happy
tummies

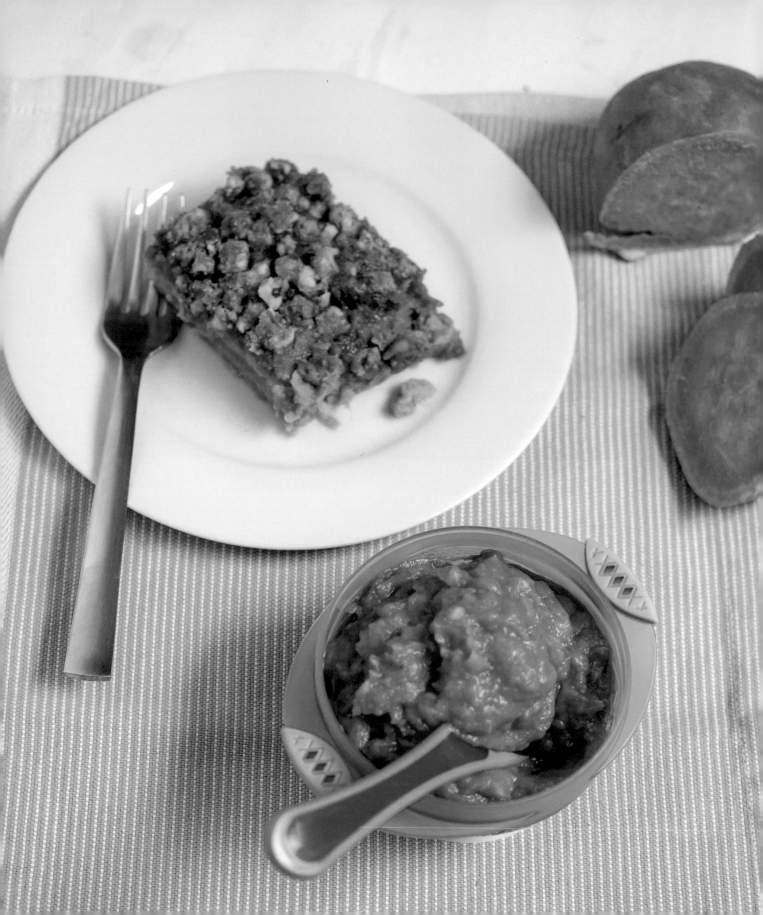

happy tummies

a cookbook for new mamas

Karen Folcik

Bright Ideas Publishing

contents

recipes

introduction

Nothing in the world compares to motherhood. For many of us, having a child creates the deepest, most honest, unconditional love we have ever felt. But that's not all. Sometimes we may also feel like we are on a roller coaster of emotions; even crazy at times.

The truth is, motherhood is wonderful and hard at the same time. We delight in playful games of peek-a-boo, and are proud to share cute photos with family and friends; yet we are tired from long sleepless nights and even longer days. We spend all our effort caring for someone else when our own needs are rarely met, and we are often uncertain about how we are performing as parents.

But through it all, we desire to be loving, affectionate, and attentive, hoping to give our little one the best start possible.

That's where this book comes in. When our babies are ready to eat solids, we want to give them the best possible nutrition. Without having fed a baby before, it may seem easiest just to buy some jars of baby food at the store. It's cooked and pureed; all you have to do is pop the lid and serve. But I'd like to show you how quick and easy it actually is to make super-healthy baby food at home. You can do it, Mama!

● ● ● ● ●

I made nearly all of my son's baby food from scratch. Not because I have endless energy or because I thought I was Supermom, but because I just fed him foods I was eating. If I had bananas at home, he had bananas. If I was making chicken and rice for dinner, that's what he had too.

This book is written for the real mom, the busy mom. It's written for you. The first section of *Happy Tummies* contains everything you need to know about starting your baby on solid foods. You'll learn the basics, like choosing the right first food, and how to go about that first feeding, as well as in-depth strategies to properly introduce new foods and textures, store and freeze baby food, and much, much more. Plus it's packed with up-to-date research and expert recommendations from organizations such as the American Academy of Pediatrics (AAP).

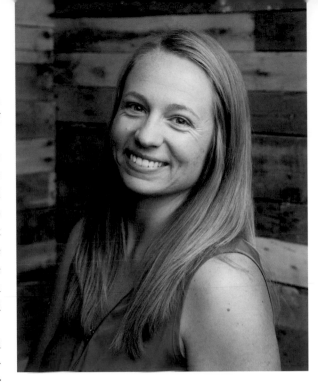

The second half of *Happy Tummies* takes over 40 whole-food ingredients and teaches you how to cook and prepare them for your baby's food so you can use what you already have at home to feed your little one. My hope is that these baby food recipes inspire you to think outside the jar, giving you the skills and confidence to craft food that is both healthy and delicious.

What's also included: nutritional information; instructions for preparing and cooking each food; recipes for the most basic purees; mix-ins to expand baby's palate; ideas for making food more exciting and nutritious; and much more. Every ingredient also features numerous recipes for parents—because we need to eat too!

No matter where you are right now on the motherhood roller coaster—whether you are eagerly anticipating your new little one, have just strapped in and arc feeling the new-mother high, or have several months under your belt—know that you have someone else (who has been there) helping you as you experience the invigorating highs, gut-wrenching lows, and confusing loop-dee-loops of parenthood. Feeding your baby wholesome food is just one more way you can help give your baby the best start possible.

Now trust yourself. Take a deep breath. And together, let's make some happy tummies.

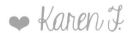

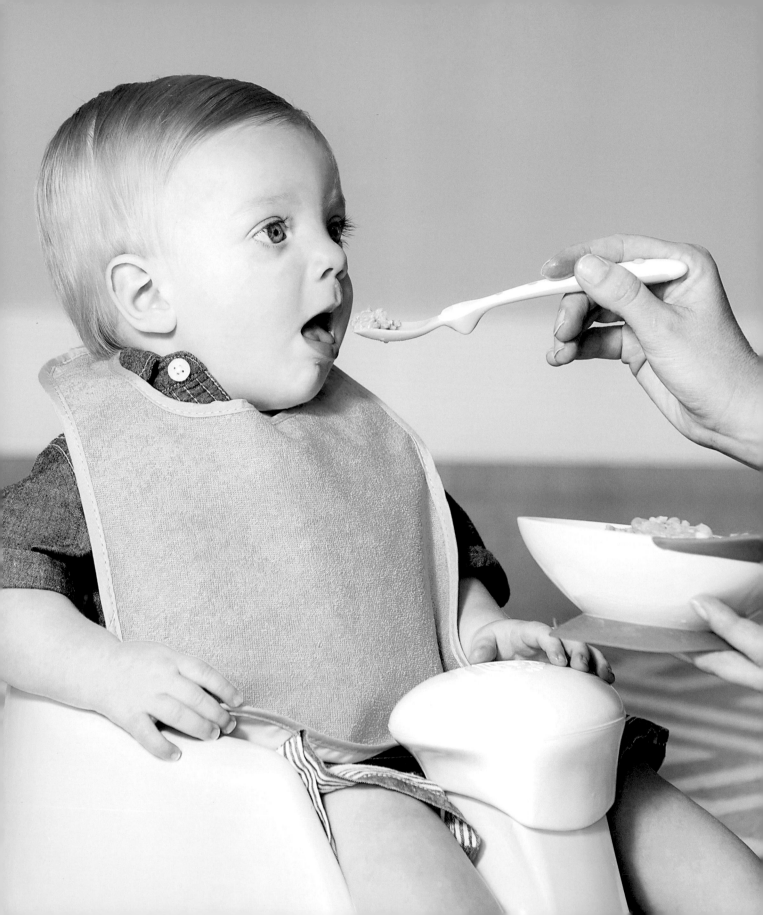

PART ONE

guidebook to feeding your baby

4 things to love about homemade baby food

1

it's the most nutritious

Most of us know that whole, natural, unprocessed foods, such as fresh fruit, vegetables, meats, and grains, are the best foods for our bodies. They are both rich in essential vitamins and nutrients and free of preservatives. Since babies may only eat a few tablespoons of food per feeding at first, they need all the nutrition they can get in each bite. By feeding baby homemade food made from the healthiest ingredients, you'll be certain that he's getting the best possible nutrition in every bite.

Commercial baby foods can work in a pinch, but you'll want to shy away from using them as your baby's sole source of solid food if you can. The methods used to process packaged foods can destroy a significant amount of the natural vitamins and nutrients, making some commercial baby food 50% less nutritious than a homemade equivalent.[1] Plus, some commercial foods contain fillers, preservatives, or unnecessary ingredients that your baby doesn't need.

2

it helps develop good eating habits

Homemade baby food is pure and simple, and tastes like its ingredients. It is the perfect first step for growing a healthy eater. Baby will learn exactly what real food tastes like. He'll get used to seeing you make his food—unpeeling a banana,

10

mashing it up, and serving it to him. He'll learn that when he's hungry, chances are you'll slice up some apple, mash up some squash, or dice some chicken. Your baby will get used to eating whole foods instead of reaching for the processed kind—and that is a good habit for you and baby!

3

experience a wide variety of textures and flavors

With your help, in just a few short months your little one will transition from eating predominantly breast milk or formula to eating table foods. You can help your baby achieve this milestone by gradually progressing the textures and flavors of his food. You'll want to start with completely smooth single-ingredient purees, move to soft, lumpy purees, and later to finely chopped table foods. Your baby will learn new skills at each stage. One of the best aspects of making homemade baby food is that you aren't stuck with just a few flavors or textures. You can completely customize your baby's food so he can try a wide variety of ingredients at the right texture.

4

saves money

Which feeding method seems more affordable? Taking a scoop out of your baked sweet potato and mashing it up for baby's dinner, or opening up a jar of store-bought sweet potato puree? If you guessed the first one, you're right! By making baby's food at home you can save a lot of money, simply by feeding baby the same thing you're already cooking up for yourself.

For those times when it's just not feasible to feed baby what everyone else is eating (ahem, pizza night), homemade food still comes out on top. One cup of homemade sweet potato puree costs me about $1.12 to make, whereas the same amount of store-bought sweet potato baby food costs about $4.16. That is a savings of 62%! Even if you add in the cost of buying a blender, you'll still save a ton of money over the long run if you make baby's food yourself.

when to start solids

Breast milk or formula with iron contains all of the nutrition your baby needs for healthy growth for the first six to nine months. Somewhere around that time—it ranges from child to child—your baby will be ready for his first taste of solid food. The process of adding solid foods to your baby's diet is called *complementary feeding*. The purpose is to teach your baby how to eat, chew, and swallow food, introduce him to a variety of flavors and textures, and provide extra nutrients that he isn't already receiving from breast milk or formula.

The general rule is to start feeding your baby solids around six months, and continue to breast or formula feed until at least one year old.[2]

The American Academy of Pediatrics (AAP) and the American Academy of Family Physicians advise not to feed your baby any food (even a taste!) before six months, because babies are not capable of handling food any earlier.[3] Doing so could cause him to choke, give him diarrhea, or even increase the risk for certain long-term diseases such as diabetes and obesity.[4] Plus, human milk is more nutritious than any kind of solid food; so for breast-fed babies, feeding too early means he'll miss out on essential nutrients and antibodies that are so good for him.[5] If your baby has any developmental delays, or you are unsure about when to start feeding solids, talk with your doctor to determine the right time.

If your baby is over six months old, and your pediatrician has given you the go-ahead, but you still aren't sure if you should start, look to your baby! Though he can't talk yet, he'll give you clues to let you know when he's ready for his first taste of solid food. He'll start eyeing your food, and maybe even reaching for it!

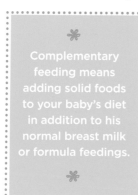

✳

Complementary feeding means adding solid foods to your baby's diet in addition to his normal breast milk or formula feedings.

✳

signs baby is ready

Before eating solid foods, your baby needs to be able to sit up in a high chair on his own and hold his head up. He also needs to have lost his tongue-thrust reflex,[7] which causes your baby to automatically push solid food out of his mouth.[8] This usually happens between four and six months.

Another sign that baby is ready for solids is that he is interested in watching you eat. He may curiously watch as you bring the loaded fork from your plate to your mouth. He may even reach for it, put his hands in his mouth, or open his mouth as if he wants you to feed him. Also, if he still seems hungry after you feed him breast milk or formula, and he's not teething or going through a growth spurt (which it would be normal for him to feed more frequently), then it may be time to start introducing solid foods.

choosing baby's first food

Infant cereal is traditionally the first food given to babies in the United States. Rice cereal mixed with breast milk, formula, or water is easy to digest, and unlikely to cause food allergies. Also, the soupy texture helps babies learn how to swallow.

Though such cereals have been recommended as the best starter food for decades, there is new

As mothers, we get lots of advice from all different sources. Friends or family members might encourage you to start feeding baby solids earlier than the recommended age. Usually it's because they aren't up to date on their information, or because that is simply what they did. Steer clear of common misconceptions like, "if you start solids early, your baby is more likely to sleep through the night" or "starting solids early helps put on weight." We know that starting solids before baby is physically ready has very little benefit and can actually be harmful.[6] If you feel that it is better for your baby to start solids early, talk to your doctor.

signs your baby is ready for solid foods

- 6–9 months old
- sits up on his own and holds his head up
- has lost his tongue-thrust reflex
- shows interest in the foods you eat
- leans forward or reaches for your food
- seems hungry after his normal feedings

research showing that infant cereals are high in carbohydrates and low in natural vitamins, minerals, and protein.[9] Though some are fortified with nutrients, infant cereal may not be the most nutritious first food.

the modern approach

In 2009 the AAP started recommending fruits, veggies, and meat in place of infant cereal for baby's first food. Finely pureed fruit, vegetables, and meat are easy to swallow and extremely nutritious. They can also help promote healthy eating preferences at a young age.[10] Despite these benefits, traditionalists argue that these foods are too advanced for young babies who may develop food allergies or have a hard time digesting.

So which is the best approach? Think about it and go with your gut. If your family has a lot of food allergies, you may want to play it safe and go with rice cereal for the first few feedings. Or if you decide on a whim that today is the day to give baby his first taste of food, and all you have at home is bananas, then go with bananas! Try to choose a food that is mild, easy to digest, and has low risk for food allergies.

Whichever you choose, this book will help you navigate the process, offering recipes on how to make your own infant cereal as well as purees that are perfect for the first feedings.

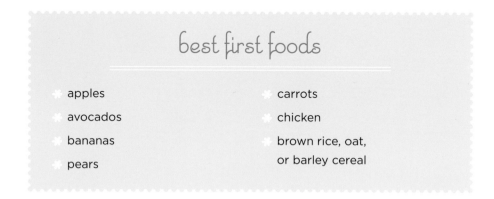

best first foods

- apples
- avocados
- bananas
- pears

- carrots
- chicken
- brown rice, oat, or barley cereal

preparing your kitchen

Baby food is so easy to make, and you only need a few simple tools to do it. You may already have everything you need! In this section you will learn what kitchen accessories are essential, how you can use what you already have, and what you can do to prepare your kitchen to cook delicious, safe baby food.

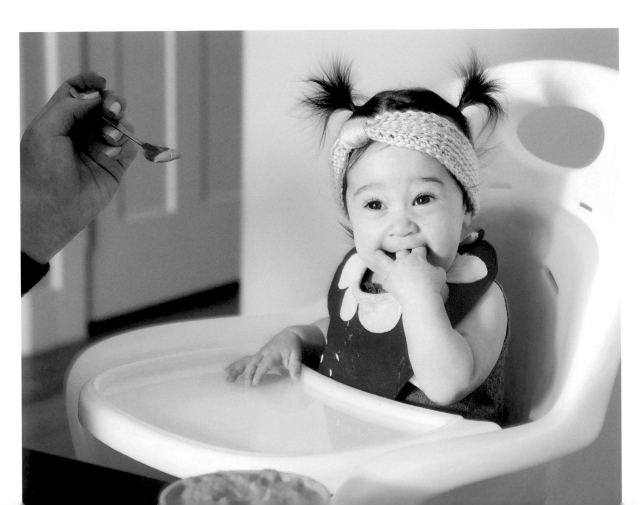

necessary kitchen tools

Here is a basic list of what you need to make your own baby food, as well as a list of items that aren't absolutely necessary, but may be helpful to have on hand. Whether you're a newbie in the kitchen or just new to making infant food, check through the list to make sure you have everything you need to get cooking.

must-haves

pureeing device: food processor, blender, fine mesh strainer, food mill, or food grinder

medium saucepan

sauté pan or nonstick skillet

colander

cutting board

spatula

measuring spoons and cups

quality knife set

soft tip or BPA-free plastic spoons

good-to-haves

roasting/baking pan

small and large saucepans

small storage containers that hold 2–4 ounces

mixing spoons

small, nonbreakable baby food bowls

flexible freezer tray with lid or freezer-safe containers

vegetable peeler

vegetable steamer

grater

permanent marker

labels for food containers

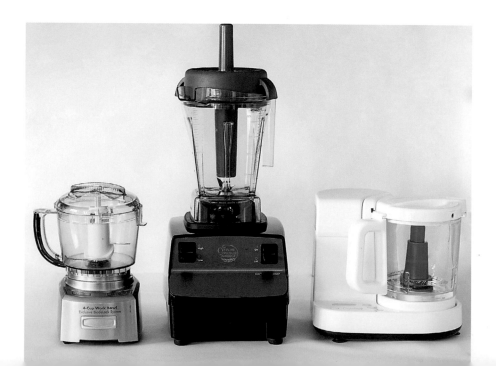

using what you have

Before you head to the store, check your cupboards to see what kitchen tools you already own. Food processors, blenders, and food mills are all excellent options for making purees.

If you don't have one of these, you can use a fork or potato masher to make a puree. It will just take a little more time and energy. Foods that don't mash up well, like chicken, you can dice up into small bits instead of pureeing.

what's the best way to puree food?

Blenders and food processors are, to me, the most helpful kitchen tools for making purees. Blenders work best for making completely smooth purees and big batches of food. They typically hold up to 9 cups, which is useful if you are making food for multiple infants or plan to do a lot of freezing. Some blenders dice and chop too. This can come in handy as you progress the texture of baby's

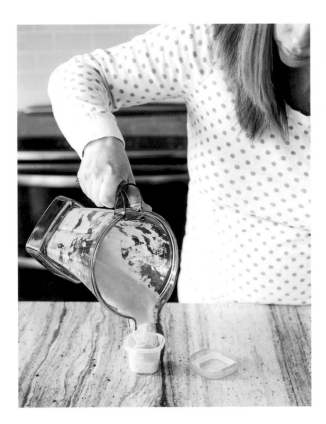
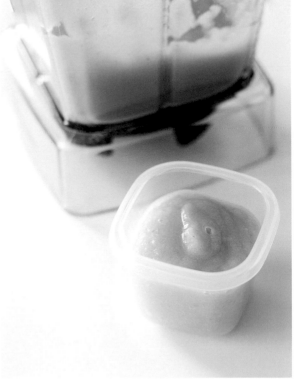

food. If you are planning to make your own infant cereal, choose one that can grind grains into flour.

Food processors are designed for dicing and chopping foods; though, many can also make purees. Use a mini food processor if you plan to make small batches of food (like most of the ones in this book).

All-in-one baby food makers are another option. These devices cook and puree food for you. Just add chopped food, choose how long to steam it, and then hit puree when it's done cooking. If you're looking for an all-in-one device, then this could be a great fit for you. Keep in mind, however, that baby food makers are typically more expensive than blenders or food processors. And you can't control the texture on many of these devices so it may only be useful for a few months.

saving money when buying kitchen equipment

Save yourself a trip and look online. You might get lucky and find a sale, an old model, or a less popular color for less money than a shiny new gadget. If you're looking for a reason to get out of the house and shop, then head straight to the clearance section to look for deals. Thrift stores, online auction sites, tag sales, and classifieds ads can all help you save some serious cash. Just be sure to give any used items a thorough cleaning before use.

preventing food poisoning

aking healthy baby food isn't just about using nutritious ingredients; it's also important to be mindful that the food you prepare is safe to eat. Babies are still developing their immune systems so they are more susceptible than adults to food poisoning.

what is food poisoning?

Food poisoning occurs when you eat food that has been contaminated by bacteria, parasites, or toxins. You can get it from unclean kitchen surfaces and utensils, unwashed fruits and vegetables, produce with a high concentration of pesticides, contaminated meats or produce, improper food storage, and more.[11]

As adults, we might not get sick at all from these things, or we might feel uncomfortable or have an upset stomach. Babies may have more severe symptoms than adults since their immune systems are so new. Call your pediatrician if you notice any symptoms of food poisoning in your infant, such as high fever, inability to keep fluids or food down, or bloody stool.

clean kitchen

By keeping a clean kitchen, you can significantly reduce the risk for food contamination. Take special care to make sure your utensils are clean before you use them, and do your best to disinfect counters after you cook.

clean fruits and vegetables properly

Food contamination can also result from unclean fruits and vegetables. To be sure your produce is clean, wash all fruits and vegetables thoroughly under cold water before cutting them. To be extra cautious, spray with a natural produce cleaner, or make your own by mixing 1 cup vinegar and 3 cups water together in a spray bottle. Spray the produce, then wash thoroughly.

wash your hands

Washing your hands regularly is another practical way to prevent foodborne illness. Hand washing strips away the bacteria, germs, and viruses that accumulate on your hands throughout the day.

Right before you start cooking, get in the habit of washing your hands with soap and hot water for 20–30 seconds. Then dry them with a clean towel. If you pick up uncooked meat, cough into your hand, touch a pet, wipe a runny nose, send a text, or just get your hands dirty somehow, give them another wash.

safe food storage

Keeping food stored properly can also help prevent food poisoning. Refrigerate all foods that can spoil, store meats separately from fruits and vegetables, and marinate foods in the refrigerator, not at room temperature.

Check that your refrigerator is set at 40° Fahrenheit (4° Celsius), and your freezer at 0° Fahrenheit (-18° Celsius). Go through your refrigerator at least once a week and throw out any food that has mold, smells off, or has expired. Wash meat and vegetable bins periodically to keep them clean.

Make sure to cover leftovers before putting them in the refrigerator, and eat them within 2–3 days. A handy rule of thumb for leftovers: If you can't remember when you cooked it, don't eat it!

tips for safe cooking

- use a clean counter

- periodically go through your refrigerator and throw out old food

- store fruits and vegetables apart from meat

- wash your hands before cooking

- don't use ingredients that look or smell bad, or have expired

- rinse fruits and vegetables even if you plan to peel them

- eat leftovers within 2-3 days

the truth about organic foods

As you begin the complementary feeding adventure, you may have some questions about what foods you should feed your little one, and in particular about whether or not you should choose *organic*. In this section, we will get to the bottom of the organic versus conventional foods debate, and discover if it really is worth buying organic.

conventional foods

Any food—fruit, vegetable, meat, poultry, egg or dairy product—that has been grown with or exposed to pesticides is considered a conventional food. Conventional growers use pesticides to prevent disease and insects, and promote better-looking, longer-lasting crops.

Conventional foods are the most common type available; it's what you can expect from your favorite restaurants and food products, unless otherwise labeled. Conventional growers are allowed to use chemical pesticides, antibiotics, chemical fertilizers, sewage sludge, ionizing radiation, and growth hormones, among other farming methods. Conventional foods may also include hotly contested genetically-engineered or modified (GMO) ingredients.

organic foods

According to the United States Department of Agriculture (USDA), foods that are grown without the use of pesticides, chemical fertilizers, or genetically modified organisms are considered organic. Animals, such as chickens, cattle, and pigs must be fed certified organic feed, and not given antibiotics or growth hormones.[12]

You can tell if a food is organic or not by its label. Usually you'll find a special sticker or label on organic food, such as "100% organic," meaning it's made entirely with organic ingredients, or "organic," meaning it's made with at least 95% organic ingredients. Some grocery stores make it easier for the organic shopper to find what they need by setting aside small sections of the store strictly for organic foods.

why it may be worth it to buy organic

Even though the US Environmental Protection Agency (EPA) sets safety limits on the amount of pesticides allowed in food, some experts suggest limiting your exposure as much as possible.[13]

Most research on the effects of pesticides on the body has been done with people who work with pesticides regularly, like conventional farmworkers. Studies have found that exposure to pesticides can cause all sorts of long-term health problems, such as asthma, autism, developmental disorders, Alzheimer's disease, nervous disorders, reproductive disorders, as well as brain, breast, and prostate cancers.[14]

pesticides and infants

Babies are particularly vulnerable to the potential health effects from pesticides because their organs and body systems are not fully developed. Pesticides stay in their bodies longer because they aren't able to metabolize and flush them out of their systems like adults.[15] They can even ingest pesticides through breast milk.[16] Since babies consume more food and liquid (compared to their body weights) than adults, there may be an elevated impact on babies.

Research has found that pesticide exposure can increase health problems for babies into toddlerhood and beyond. One study found that boys 8–15 years old were twice as likely to develop ADHD when they were exposed to a common household pesticide.[17] Three other studies found that pesticides may increase the risk for developmental delays and autism among kids by as much as 25%.[18] Another study found that children scored lower on IQ tests when their mothers had high levels of pesticides in their bodies during pregnancy.[19]

Though the research on the effects of eating food treated with pesticides is lacking, what we can draw from other research is that pesticide exposure can have a big impact on the development of our little ones, and on our overall health.

lessening pesticides in your diet

Some pesticides are absorbed into food, such as in fruits and vegetables, whereas others remain on the surface. For some produce, like potatoes and carrots, you can simply peel or wash them and instantly reduce your exposure to pesticides. For many foods, however, the pesticides cannot be easily removed.

One obvious way to lessen the amount of pesticides in your diet is to choose organic food whenever possible. In a Consumer Reports study that tested pesticides in a variety of organic and conventional fruits and vegetables, organic produce was found to have significantly less pesticides.[20] Another study by the University of Washington School of Public Health found that people who ate organic diets had significantly less pesticides in their bodies than those who ate conventional foods. Another study found that people who ate mostly organic foods had 89% less pesticide residue in their bodies.[21] Organic food contains less pesticides than conventional foods, and for some, that's enough to believe it's the healthier, safer food option.

produce with the most and least pesticides

Every year the Environmental Working Group comes out with a list of the fruits and vegetables that tend to have the highest and lowest exposures to pesticides. Snap a picture of this list with your phone so you have it with you at the grocery store, or download the EWG's Dirty Dozen smartphone app.[22]

the dirtiest foods (shop organic)

apples	spinach
peaches and nectarines	cucumbers
strawberries	tomatoes
grapes	snap peas
celery	potatoes

the cleanest foods (buy conventional)

avocados	kiwifruits
sweet corn	onions
pineapples	asparagus
papayas	cantaloupe
mangos	cauliflower

the gist

The best nutrition you can give your family is a healthy diet of fruits, vegetables, grains, and proteins, regardless of whether or not they are organic or conventional. Though there is little evidence that organic food is more nutritious, eating organic can help your family create a healthier lifestyle and lessen your exposure to disease-causing pesticides.

If you haven't been choosing organic, don't panic! There is evidence that young kids can detoxify quickly from harmful chemicals. A 2006 study found that when children switched to an organic diet, the levels of pesticides in their bodies dropped so significantly that they were no longer detectable.[23]

So if you don't already buy organic foods, you may want to start. Even small changes, like choosing just a handful of organically grown produce every time you shop, can help to protect your family from pesticides. And if you can, start your baby on organic foods from the beginning.

practical tips for buying organic

Organic food does tend to be more expensive than conventional food. To save money, try these tips:

* **buy organic meat in bulk.** If your grocery store offers organic meat in a big pack, choose that and freeze what you don't plan to use right away.

* **check out the frozen food section.** Often, organic fruit and vegetables are more affordable frozen than fresh.

* **select an assortment of organic and conventional food products.** Try to focus on buying organic dairy products and meat, as well as the fruits and vegetables with the highest exposure to pesticides. Buy conventional for the rest.

* **focus on what your family eats the most.** For example, if your family eats more chicken than beef, splurge on organic chicken and buy conventional beef.

* **choose generic brands instead of name brands.** Many grocers make their own lines of organic products. They are usually good quality and more affordable than name brands.

* **shop around.** Look at local, discount, and health food stores, to see where you can find the best prices. Subscribe to store newsletters to see what's on sale.

* **if you can't swing it for the whole family, buy organic just for baby's food.**

cooking baby's food

The first step to making homemade baby food is cooking the ingredients. Nearly all food requires cooking before being pureed. Even fruit, like apples and peaches, should be cooked first for easier digestion. Cooking also makes food softer so it's easier to puree.

Cook fruits, vegetables, and grains until they are very tender, and cook all meats until they are well-done. Since foods and appliances vary, use the cooking times in this book as a guideline, and check your food regularly to be sure it's cooking properly. Let food cool so it's just slightly warm or room temperature before feeding baby.

introducing new foods

For the first month, try cooking single-ingredient purees or cereals, such as apple puree or infant rice cereal. This helps keep the flavors basic and limits food allergies. Feed baby the same food for several meals over several days before introducing him to another food appropriate for his age. Check out the age guide for introducing solid foods on page 246 to help you choose foods appropriate for each age.

Over a period of a few months, introduce baby to a wide variety of fruits, vegetables, meats, and grains. As a general guideline, wait a few days between offering new foods to give you time to spot a food allergy and give baby time to get used to the new food.

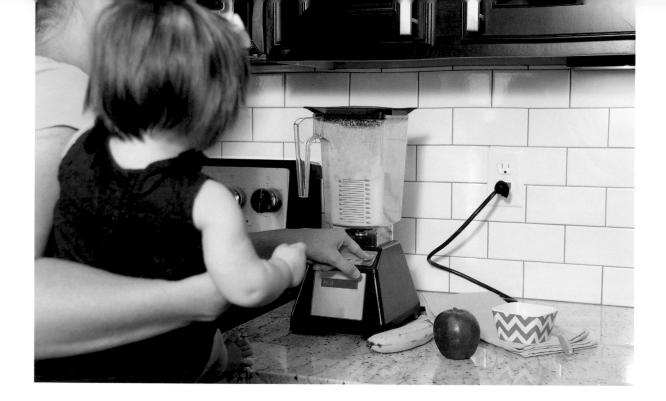

making tasty baby food

Baby food doesn't have to be bland or boring! Once baby has been introduced to a couple different ingredients on their own, you can start to mix foods for more complex flavors. Try blending foods within the same food category—fruits with other fruits and vegetables with other vegetables. Or try mixing foods of different categories, like meats with vegetables, or fruits with grains.

The recipes in this this book show how easy it is to mix flavors and make delicious tasting baby food. For each ingredient you'll learn how to prepare and cook a basic puree. You'll also find recipes for mix-ins to help you make tasty and exciting homemade baby food.

flavor boosting cooking methods

You'll also learn different methods of cooking—like roasting and grilling—to create flavor. Roasting, the process of cooking at a high temperature in the oven, causes ingredients to brown, caramelizing or creating a crust, which adds more flavor to most foods. Grilling adds a slightly smoky flavor. By branching out and trying different cooking methods, you can introduce baby to new tastes and enhance the flavor of his favorite foods.

guidebook to feeding your baby

preserve nutrients during cooking

Choose steaming, sautéing, roasting, grilling, or broiling over boiling foods whenever possible. Boiling can cause nutrients from the food to leak into the water, making the food less nutritious. If you do choose to boil, save some of the water from the pot and use it as the liquid to thin purees. This will help restore some of the lost nutrients.

purees to finger foods

Progressing the texture of baby's food helps him become a confident, skilled eater. Start out by preparing smooth, soupy purees. Once he's gotten used to that texture, advance to slightly thicker but still smooth purees. As your baby gets better at swallowing and chewing, continue progressing the texture of his food. Move on to soft purees with tiny lumps, like mashed potatoes. Then introduce ground foods, like ground beef. Within just a few months, he'll graduate from smooth purees to soft, finely chopped finger foods.

should I add salt, sugar, or seasoning to baby's food?

The AAP suggests waiting until baby is at least 12 months before adding any salt, sugar, or seasoning to his food. This helps your baby learn what food tastes like naturally, and can contribute to healthy eating preferences later on.

helpful hints

* always start with ripe fruit and vegetables for best results. Using unripe fruit will alter the taste and texture of the baby food.

* thaw frozen fruit in the refrigerator overnight or in the microwave if you'll be cooking and serving it right away

* don't re-freeze food that has already been frozen

* cook fruit, vegetables, and grains until very tender and meat until well-done

* keep a bag of frozen vegetables in the freezer for an easy heat, puree, and serve baby meal

* make infant cereal for younger babies and grains in their whole form if you want to add some texture

baby food texture chart

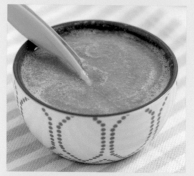

Below are general guidelines to help you progress baby's food. This chart is particularly helpful when making your own baby food recipes. All of the baby food recipes in this book have age guidelines to help you advance the texture of baby's food. Use these as general references, modifying the texture as needed for your baby.

6 months old: smooth, soupy, one ingredient puree

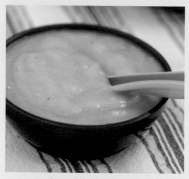

7 months old: smooth, soupy, combination ingredient puree

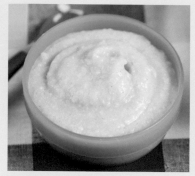

8 months old: smooth, thicker puree

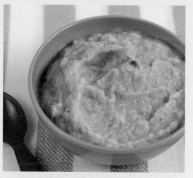

9 months old: soft puree with tiny soft lumps

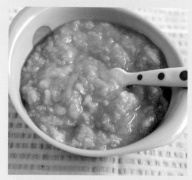

10 months old: soft, mashed puree with lumps, ground, or finely chopped soft foods

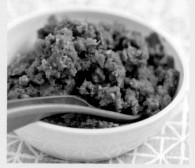

11 months old: finely chopped soft foods, mashed foods

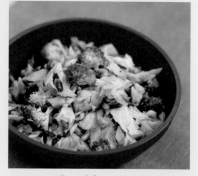

12 months old: baby bite-sized pieces of food

foods to avoid

By the time baby is 12 months, nearly all foods are safe to eat as long as they are the right texture. Before his first birthday, there are just a few foods to avoid:

junk food!

The goal of complementary feeding is to help baby learn to eat real food and give him supplemental nutrition. Since babies have such small bellies, giving them any kind of junk food fills them up with empty calories without any of the nutrition your baby needs. Avoid feeding baby high calorie foods like cookies and cakes. Not even one bite! And avoid salty foods like french fries or chips, and sugary drinks like fruit juice or soda.

cow's milk

Breast milk and formula are the healthiest drinks for babies. Wait on cow's milk until after baby is twelve months old; he won't be able to process this type of milk any earlier. Cow's milk can irritate your baby's intestines or cause a food allergy. And it doesn't provide the right nutrition for infants.

Other types of dairy, like small amounts of cheese, cottage cheese, or yogurt, are easier to digest, and are okay to feed babies nine months old and up.

choking hazards

Always keep a close eye on baby when he eats. A choking baby may not be able to cry or make a noise, so if you are in the next room or he is in his car seat, it's possible that baby could choke and you wouldn't know. Even pureed foods can cause a new eater to choke if he has too much in his mouth or has a tough time swallowing.

When you choose finger foods for baby, make sure they are small and soft. Avoid any potential choking hazards, like meat with bones, big pieces of food, chunks of cheese, raw vegetables, marshmallows, gum, nuts, whole grapes, or anything else that is noticeably tough to chew.

honey

Wait until baby is at least twelve months old to offer honey, as it can sometimes cause infant botulism. Botulism is a potentially fatal gastrointestinal illness caused by bacteria that more mature immune systems can handle.

Avoid feeding baby any kind of shellfish, like lobster, clams, shrimp, mussels, and crab, as it could cause a food allergy. Low-mercury fish, such as salmon and tilapia, however, are safe to introduce to babies six months and up.

You may want to go over this list with all of your baby's caretakers, including grandparents and babysitters, to help them understand what they can feed baby. It may seem obvious to you as a parent, but to temporary caretakers, a cookie with a cup of milk or fast food fries might seem like a fine snack.

identifying food allergies

Food allergies occur when the body has an immune response to an ingredient. Identifying food allergies in adults can be tricky because we eat such a wide variety of foods, so it can be tough to pinpoint what's causing our discomfort. If you introduce new foods slowly and as single ingredients, it should be easier to identify what's causing a food allergy for an infant.

common allergenic foods

Cow's milk, egg whites, peanuts and tree nuts, fish, shellfish, soy, and wheat are the most common allergenic foods for babies.

Traditionally, experts have recommended waiting to feed babies any food that may cause a food allergy. Some recent research, however, has found that introducing babies to allergenic foods early on may actually protect him from ever developing an allergy.[24] You may want to talk with your pediatrician before introducing your child to a typically allergenic food.

symptoms

Symptoms of food allergies—from mild to severe—can present immediately or hours after eating. They may show up every time baby eats the allergenic food, or just if he has a lot of it. Food allergies can also develop over time. A baby is at a higher risk of developing a food allergy if his parents or siblings have the same food-related problem. If you are worried that your baby could have food allergies, talk with your doctor.

You can tell your baby is having a mild allergic reaction if he gets diarrhea or a rash, has a noticeable increase in gas, or is extremely fussy during or after he eats. If your baby has one of these symptoms, stop feeding him solids and try to relieve his symptoms. Offer to nurse if you are breastfeeding. Once baby is feeling better, think about the foods you have fed him in the past few days. Don't feed him anything that you suspect could be the cause of the allergy, and talk with your doctor.

If your baby gets hives, has facial swelling, or trouble breathing, he may be having a severe allergic reaction. Call 911 or go to the hospital for immediate medical attention.

If your baby has any signs of food allergies, make sure to write it down. We have busy lives and it can be hard to recall exactly what foods have caused allergies or what symptoms developed. Record any suspected food allergies in the food allergy journal on page 249.

the most common signs of food allergies in infants[4]

- face, tongue, or lip swelling
- eczema or hives
- rash
- asthma or sneezing
- fussiness while eating

- difficulty breathing or wheezing
- loss of consciousness in extreme cases
- diarrhea or vomiting
- rash around the anus or gassiness

the first feeding

You've been anticipating it, and now it's finally time! Try to think of baby's first time eating solids as more of a *taste* than a feeding or a meal. Sit baby on your lap and put a little bit of the food on the tip of your finger or soft-tipped spoon. Then put it near his mouth. Let him lean over and taste the food. You can keep adding a little more food to your finger or spoon until he doesn't want any more. Next time casually feed him from your lap again or put him in an infant chair or high chair and feed him with a spoon, whichever feels more comfortable.

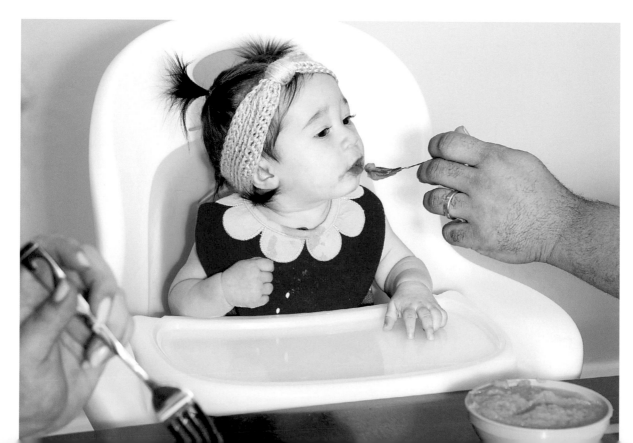

step-by-step guide to feeding baby solids

step 1

Choose a time of the day when you aren't in a hurry and are in a good mood. Sometimes baby's first feeding can go well. Maybe he'll try it and smile, or maybe he'll spit it out or make a mess. However it goes, try to make sure you have the time and patience to be supportive of your little one as he tries something new. A smile or some words of encouragement can go a long way.

step 2

To start, put a small amount of pureed food or infant cereal in a small bowl. Sit your baby on your lap and put a bib on him.

step 3

Test the food to make sure it is lukewarm or room temperature. Then put about a half teaspoon or less on the tip of your finger or a spoon.

> *
> Placing baby on your lap helps him feel safe and secure as he tries something entirely new. Your loving support as you introduce him to food can help strengthen your mother-baby bond, and teach him that meals are a time for family to come together.
> *

Your washed finger is a great utensil for the first taste because baby is already very familiar with your body. (He's probably already used to gnawing on your fingers!) Plus, your finger is warm and soft. If using a spoon, choose one with a rubber tip, or one that's made entirely of BPA-free plastic. Plastic is softer than metal in baby's mouth.

step 4

Move your finger or spoon towards baby's mouth, and wait for him to open it. When he shows you he's ready, place your finger or spoon right near his mouth and let him close on the food.

step 5

Watch his reaction and smile. Your baby just had his first bite of solid food! All babies are different, so don't worry if he spits it out or just lets the food sit on his tongue. With practice your baby will learn how to swallow and chew.

If baby gets upset or turns his head when you offer the spoon, it could mean he's not ready. Don't force it. Go back to exclusively breastfeeding or formula feeding for a week or so and try again later.

step 6

Continue feeding baby until he is full or doesn't want any more. He may be done after one or two tastes.

step 7

Throw away any leftover food that your finger, spoon, or the baby touched. Congratulations, you just completed your first solid food feeding! Great job, Mama!

how much to feed baby

When baby first starts eating solid foods, aim to feed once a day, and offer about 1–2 teaspoons of food per feeding. Gradually increase to two feedings with more food each time; follow your baby's lead. Continue to breastfeed or formula feed, as this provides the majority of your baby's nutrition. Generally, by around 8 or 9 months, babies naturally increase solid feedings to three times a day.

baby cues

Learning your baby's cues for when he is still hungry or full will help you feed him the right amount of food. Allow him to eat until he is full, and try to avoid forcing him to eat "just one more bite," or finish all that you prepared. Doing so teaches him that he isn't actually full when his body tells him that he is, and can lead to overeating later in life.[26]

On the other hand, restricting food for fear that baby will overeat is equally unhealthy.[27] Allow baby to eat until he is satisfied. This will help him develop healthy eating patterns and a healthy relationship with food.

Look for long, wide bibs with a crumb tray or pocket. These are an excellent investment. They will be useful for several months as baby transitions from purees to finger foods. For super messy eaters, consider a bib smock—a bib that you slide on over baby's arms and chest. This bib offers full coverage to keep his outfit clean during meals.

guidebook to feeding your baby

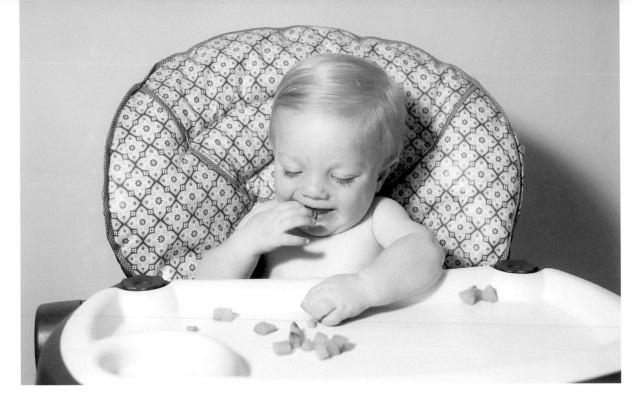

independent feeders

Some babies prefer to feed themselves. Grated apples, small chunks of cooked potato, bits of shredded meat, such as chicken or pork, and ground beef or ground turkey are great first finger foods.

To teach baby to self-feed, just put a few pieces of food in front of him. Let him pick it up and eat at his own pace. Continue to add more pieces to his tray until he no longer brings food to his mouth.

how to tell when your baby is:

FULL	STILL HUNGRY
turns his head away from the food	shows an interest in continuing to eat
pushes away the spoon	opens mouth for food
seals his lips together	puts hands in mouth
pushes food out of his mouth	is excited and happy

Depending on what you are having for dinner, you may find it easier to spoon feed purees for some meals, and give baby little bits of food for others. Babies as young as six months are capable of self-feeding. Just be sure to supervise the entire time.

food play

Babies love to play with their food. And though it's messy, allowing him to do so is actually good for his sensory development. Purees are like edible finger paint to a baby. Small bits of food are fun to eat, smoosh, and throw. Allowing baby to explore with his hands helps him learn what food looks, smells, tastes, and feels like. It also helps teach him the differences between food and non-food substances.

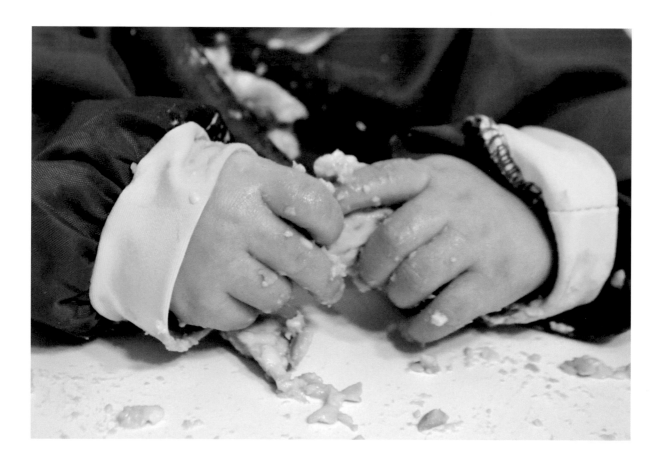

If you are spoon-feeding baby, and he wants to participate, hand him a spoon to play with. He learns by watching you. Playing chug-a-chug-a-choo and airplane spoon promotes bonding and helps teach baby that mealtime can be fun.

control the mess

Mess is inevitable at all stages of the feeding process. What you'll need to figure out is how best to control or clean up the mess while still allowing baby to explore his food.

mealtime mats

The first option is prevention. Most baby stores sell vinyl or plastic mats that you can put under a high chair to protect your floor from spills and stains. There are also disposable mats, and ones that can be tossed in the washing machine and used multiple times. These are really helpful if you don't want to mop your floor after each feeding. Dried purees harden like concrete on tile floors and can stain carpets. These mats can help make life a little bit easier.

hand-held vacuum

When baby is eating chunky purees or finger foods, you may find that a cordless, hand-held vacuum becomes your new best friend. As babies get older, they delight in games, such as throwing food off their high chairs. Hand-held vacuums are light and efficient. Keep one plugged in on the counter for easy access.

storing and freezing homemade baby food

Since babies only eat a small amount per feeding, you will likely get multiple meals out of each batch of baby food. Any food that hasn't been touched by your baby or his spoon, and hasn't been out on the counter for two or more hours, can be safely stored away. Leftover baby food stays fresh in the refrigerator for one or two days, and up to three months in the freezer.

choosing the right container

Though you probably already have a bunch of containers for storing leftovers, you may want to consider getting some specifically for baby food. It can be helpful to put your baby's food in tiny, colorful containers because they will be portioned into servings, and stand out in the refrigerator among all the other food and containers. When choosing containers, check to make sure they are BPA- and phthalate-free and have tight fitting lids. Below are some of the most popular types of baby food containers.

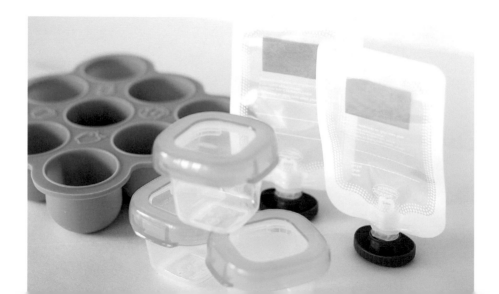

If you plan to freeze leftovers, you'll want to use a container that is specifically marked *freezer-safe*. Freezer-safe containers keep food fresh and retain natural moisture, color, flavor, and texture. When possible, avoid plastic wrap, wax paper, and regular containers and bags that aren't labeled freezer-safe. These products won't protect the food for long-term storage. You don't want to end up with freezer burn!

jars and cubes

Small plastic jars or cubes are great for storing baby food. They are easy to use and usually work well in both the refrigerator and freezer. Jars and cubes specifically made for baby food come in plastic, silicone, or glass. Choose ones that hold 2–4 ounces of food, are labeled chemical-free, and have a leak-proof seal. Avoid any jar that comes with a metal lid because the liner may contain BPA.

freezer trays

For large batches of baby food, you may want to consider a freezer tray. These look like ice cube trays, with several small cubes attached. Just pour your puree into the cubes, cover, and freeze. When you need a serving, just pop out one of the servings, and put the rest back in the freezer.

Choose a freezer tray with a tightly fitting lid so that it also works as a storage container. You can use a freezer tray temporarily without a lid, but once frozen you'll need to pop out the servings and store long-term in a freezer-safe bag.

Freezer trays come in plastic, silicone, and stainless steel, but the silicone trays are the easiest for pushing out frozen food. Typically, one cube equals 2 tablespoons of food.

squeeze pouch

Squeeze pouches have dual purposes. They store food and also allow baby to eat independently. Instead of spoon-feeding, baby sucks the food directly from the pouch. This is convenient for the occasional on-the-go snack, but try to use it sparingly. Babies need to learn to spoon and finger feed in order to develop their eating skills, so it's not recommended to use squeeze pouches as a primary method, especially for younger babies.

If you want to use squeeze pouches as containers for homemade baby food, choose the one-time-use kind. The reusable ones can be tough to clean. Pouches with large spouts or kits that come with a filler tube make it easier to fill. Squeeze pouches are usually both refrigerator and freezer-safe, and hold about 4 ounces of baby food.

freezing baby food

Making baby food ahead of time and storing it in the freezer is an excellent way to save time and energy. Who couldn't use more of that? It can be lifesaving to have a few homemade "freezer meals" for baby on those tiresome days when you just need to have Chinese take-out or pizza for dinner.

Prepping food for the freezer is easy! Just make a batch of food and let it cool. Choose a freezer-safe storage container and label it with the name of the food and the date. Use the frozen food within three months and check that your freezer is set to at least 0° Fahrenheit. Never re-freeze food. Once it's thawed, either use it or throw it away.

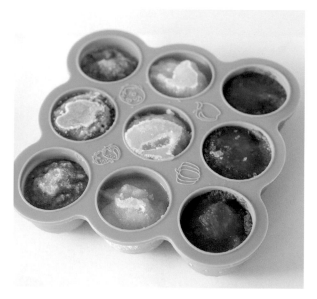
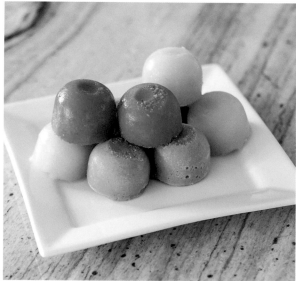

guidebook to feeding your baby

how to freeze baby food using . . .

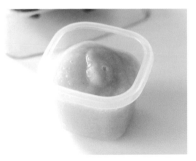 **small jars:** Pour the puree in the container, leaving some room at the top to allow for the liquid to expand. Label it with the contents and date. Cover, then pop it in the freezer.

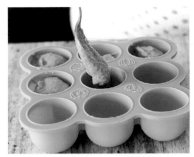 **a freezer tray:** Spoon the puree into the cubes, cover, and freeze. If you're using a freezer tray without a lid, or a standard ice cube tray, pour the puree into the cubes, cover with plastic wrap, then freeze. Once frozen, pop out the food and put it in a freezer bag or freezer-safe container. Label with the contents and date.

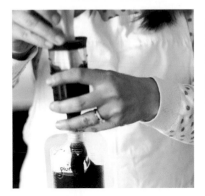 **squeeze pouches:** Fill the pouch with baby food, leaving some room at the top of the pouch. Try to squeeze the air out of the pouch without squeezing out the food. Seal it up, label it, and place it in the freezer.

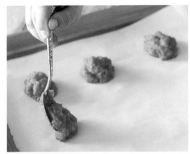 **a cookie sheet:** Line a cookie sheet with wax paper. Spoon small portions of baby food a few inches apart on the cookie sheet. Freeze, then use a spatula to transfer the food into a freezer-safe bag or container. Label it with the contents and date. Pop it back in the freezer.

reheat frozen baby food safely

Frozen baby food just needs to be warmed up. If you're defrosting a food that you would normally serve cold, like apple puree, then just warm it to room temperature. Here are a few options for safely reheating frozen food:

bowl of water method: Place the jar, pouch, or sealed plastic bag in a bowl of warm water to thaw and warm the food. This should take about 10–20 minutes. Remove when the food is warm.

stovetop method: For use with the jar, freezer tray, or cookie sheet methods, scoop the food out of the container and place it in a small saucepan. Heat on medium-low until warmed. Test to make sure the food isn't too hot before feeding it to baby.

microwave method: Although you can reheat food in the microwave, it's not recommended. Microwaving creates hot spots, meaning some parts are scalding hot, while others may still be cool.

For use with the jar, freezer tray, or cookie sheet methods only, scoop the food into a microwave-safe bowl, then nuke until warm. Stir, stir, stir, and stir some more to help eliminate hot spots. Then test the temperature of the food, feeding baby only when it's lukewarm.

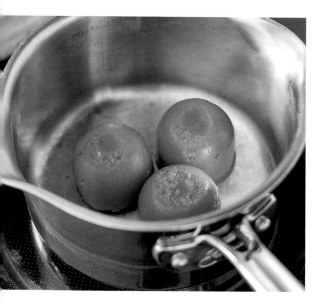
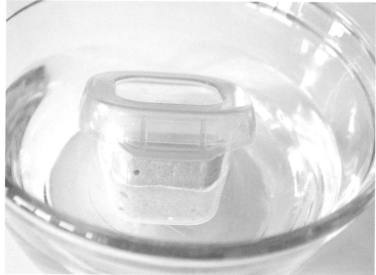

42

balancing breastfeeding or formula feeding

As you already know, your baby will get the majority of his nutrition from breast milk or formula until he is one year old. Solid food is just an additional form of nourishment for baby. During this first year, continue your normal feeding schedule while slowly adding solid foods so he gets used to the taste and texture of food.

breastfeeding FAQs

When should I stop breastfeeding?

Breastfeeding can be demanding at times, but many moms find that it gets easier the longer they go. Not only does breastfeeding build a strong bond between you and your baby, it also has significant health benefits for you both and your baby. Evidence-based research has found that babies who are breastfed past four months tend to be significantly healthier than those who are weaned earlier. Breastfed babies have a lower risk of developing: allergies, diabetes, childhood cancers, celiac disease, GI infections, SIDS, respiratory tract infections, obesity in adolescence and adulthood and more. There is also an abundance of evidence that breastfeeding significantly boosts childhood IQ scores.[28]

Breastfeeding for six months or longer may have health benefits for you, too. Mothers who exclusively breastfeed past six months tend to have lower blood pressure, and fewer instances of heart disease, diabetes, breast, and ovarian cancers.

Even after starting solid foods, breast milk is still extremely nutritious and valuable. It can provide at least half of all of your baby's nutrients from 6–12 months. If you choose to keep breastfeeding after one year, it can provide up to one-third of your baby's nutrition.[29]

The AAP recommends breastfeeding babies until they are at least one year old[30]; though, other sources such as the World Health Organization[31] and UNICEF[32] recommend at least two years. Despite these recommendations, nurse as long as you and your baby want to continue. You may have already stopped breastfeeding, or you may want to nurse through toddlerhood. Only you and your baby know when when it's the right time to wean.

Will I run out of milk once I start to feed baby solid foods?

Milk production works on a supply-and-demand basis. Your body will keep up with your baby's nursing schedule and produce as much milk as he normally drinks. If your baby feeds frequently, your body will start making more milk right after each nursing session because it knows that your baby will want to eat again soon after. As your baby eats more solid foods and nurses less, your body will slowly decrease supply.

As long as you keep expressing milk, either via breastfeeding or with a pump, your body will continue to make it. You can even keep breastfeeding when your child is a toddler, and eats three meals a day plus snacks, if you express regularly.

For more information on breastfeeding, find a local La Leche League support group or read their guide, *The Womanly Art of Breastfeeding*. Lactation counselors can also be extremely helpful. They are certified to provide counseling, education, and support. They are mothers who have successfully breastfed their own children, so they often bring personal experience to other breastfeeding mamas. With a quick Internet search you'll likely find many lactation counselors in your area.

Should I use breast milk to thin purees?

If you have extra breast milk and are already pumping, then go for it! Adding breast milk to baby's purees will make the food even more nutritious. Otherwise, use filtered water to thin purees.

formula feeding FAQs

When should I stop formula feeding?

Like with breastfeeding, continue formula feeding through baby's first birthday to ensure he is getting the nutrition he needs. Beyond the first year, there is no set time at which you should transition to whole milk or water.

Should I cut back the amount of formula he's drinking when I introduce solid foods?

Keep your baby on the same feeding schedule when you introduce solids, since formula will supply most of his nutrition during his first year. Don't, however, force him to finish his bottle if he's not hungry.

Should I start feeding baby water or juice when he starts solids?

It's okay to offer up to 8 ounces of filtered water a day to keep your formula-fed baby hydrated. Try to wait until your baby is a toddler before introducing juice, as it is sugary and could shape his young tastes to prefer juice instead of water.

Is it okay to add cereal to baby's bottle?

No. Pediatricians don't recommend adding cereal to baby's bottle, unless they find it medically necessary. When baby is ready for solids, put a little food on your finger or on a spoon, and offer it to baby that way.

Should I use water or formula to thin baby's purees?

Commercially prepared infant formula will add more vitamins and nutrients, but water will work just fine to thin purees.

ask the nutritionist

assandra Edwards, MS, Registered and Licensed Dietitian, answers some of your most commonly asked questions.

What do I do if my baby starts to choke?

Sometimes when babies are eating, they will gag and spit up their food. This is all a part of learning how to eat. It's normal. Just sit with baby to make sure he's okay. However, if baby chokes and is having trouble breathing, call for emergency services. Take baby out of his high chair and lay him on your arm facedown. Place him so that his head is slightly lower than his body and firmly pat the middle of his back with the heel of your other hand until the food is dislodged.

It is always a good idea to take a course in infant first aid and safety. Consider downloading a phone app, such as *First Aid* by American Red Cross, and reviewing emergency steps every few months.

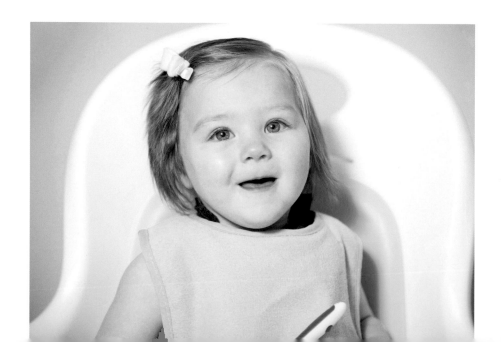

Should I feed baby solid foods every day?

Introducing solids is as much about learning to eat and learning about food as it is about getting appropriate nutrition. Just like learning anything else, practice makes perfect, and once baby is ready to start solids, it is ideal to offer solids every day.

When should I start feeding baby two meals a day? What about three?

Let your baby be your guide. The first few days that you offer solid foods, feed him once a day during the same meal, for example, every day at breakfast. Once baby is accepting food and shows interest, start offering it twice, and then three times a day. You might notice that when you sit down for a meal, baby is very interested in your food. If so, feel free to offer baby food that is appropriate. By 7–8 months, baby will probably be eating several tablespoons of food three times a day.

Is it okay to cook baby's food in butter or oil?

Healthy fats are essential for baby's brain development. Remember that moderation is key and too much of a good thing can quickly turn into a bad thing. But parents don't need to be afraid to give their babies a little fat either.

Baby's first tastes should be single foods rather than mixed dishes. If an allergic reaction occurs, this makes the culprit easier to identify. For this reason, steer clear of adding butter or oils to those first foods. After baby has had a single food, go ahead and add a little butter or oil during cooking. For example, if baby has had plain carrots several times with no problem, add a little butter to the carrots. Grass-fed butter, canola oil, olive oil, and high-oleic safflower oil are examples of healthy fats.

When does baby need to eat from all five food groups during the day?

When baby is weaned from breast milk or formula completely, all nutrition must be supplied from solids. This requires a diet that includes all food groups. This milestone will occur at different times for different babies, but around twelve months is common.

Can baby eat meat that has been cooked in sauce, like a stew?

Sauce is okay for your baby, and could actually help him chew and swallow meat better. Younger babies who are just starting solids still need to start with single

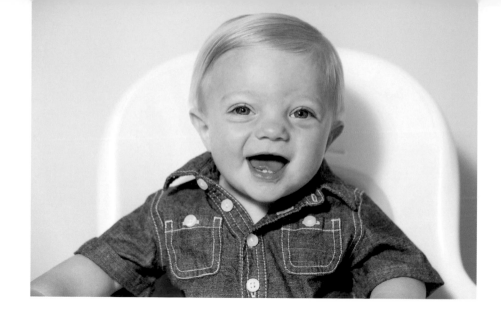

foods. If your baby has had the meat several times before with no problems, serving with sauce would be the next step.

Will my milk production decrease when baby starts to eat solid foods?

Yes. Milk production works on a supply and demand system; the more baby demands, the more Mommy supplies. During the first few months that baby receives solid food, it is more about learning to eat than about getting nutrition from food. Your baby probably won't be eating enough food to affect his demand much, so at first you might not notice a difference in milk supply. Once the solid food meals grow a little larger, your baby will demand less milk. You might notice that your breasts feel less full and that you pump less volume.

I've noticed some changes in baby's poop since he started eating solid foods. Is that normal?

What goes in must come out, and no one pays more attention to the in and the out than a mom. The color, consistency, and odor reflect what baby is eating and sometimes give clues about health issues. Moms are often alarmed when poop changes. But you can expect that any time baby's diet changes, his poop will also change.

Poop of an exclusively breastfed baby is drastically different from poop of an exclusively formula-fed baby, but after solids are introduced, the poop is not so different. The poop of your exclusively breastfed baby will change from mushy, yellow/green with a sweet smell to brown and mushy (but thicker) with an offensive odor. Your formula-fed infant's poop will go from brown, sticky, and slightly offensive in odor to thicker and darker with a more offensive odor.

You may also notice chunks of undigested food from time to time, or hard clumps when your baby starts eating solids. These are both normal unless either become increasingly more frequent. If this happens, it is a good idea to check in with your doctor. Also, call your doctor if you notice either fresh blood (bright red) or dried blood (black) in baby's poop.

What should I feed baby when he has a cold?

When babies are sick, they can be rather selective with their foods, just like adults. Because babies are still learning how to coordinate eating solids, swallowing, and breathing, an excessive amount of mucus in their sinuses and throat can make it difficult to eat and and could make them nauseated. Many times this comes with a sore, swollen throat, which makes eating more painful and difficult. Let baby eat what he can and is willing to eat. If he has a sore throat, he might have a preference for cold or warm foods. Everyone is different.

Foods that are thinner and softer like soup, noodles, and mashed vegetables might be accepted better than harder solids, like diced fruit and crackers. Continue to offer a wide variety of foods that include protein, fruit, and vegetables, which are full of nutrition to help baby heal faster.

What is this craze about feeding babies probiotics? Are there any real benefits?

Healthy gut bacteria accounts for a large portion of the human immune system. In other words, we need those good bugs in our tummies to protect us and keep us healthy. Sometimes, illness, medication, and exposure to other substances kill off those good bugs and allow more of the bad bugs to grow. You can treat this by filling the gut with more of the good guys (through probiotics) and feeding those good guys (through prebiotics). The community of good bugs and bad bugs that set up camp in your tummy is known as the gut microbiome. The microbiome is a hot topic right now.

Whether or not your baby needs more probiotics depends on their environment and health and is something to discuss with your doctor. Fermented foods like kimchi naturally provide probiotics. Prebiotics come from foods like bananas and legumes. But before you stuff your little one with kimchi and beans, remember that balance is important. Don't over do it.

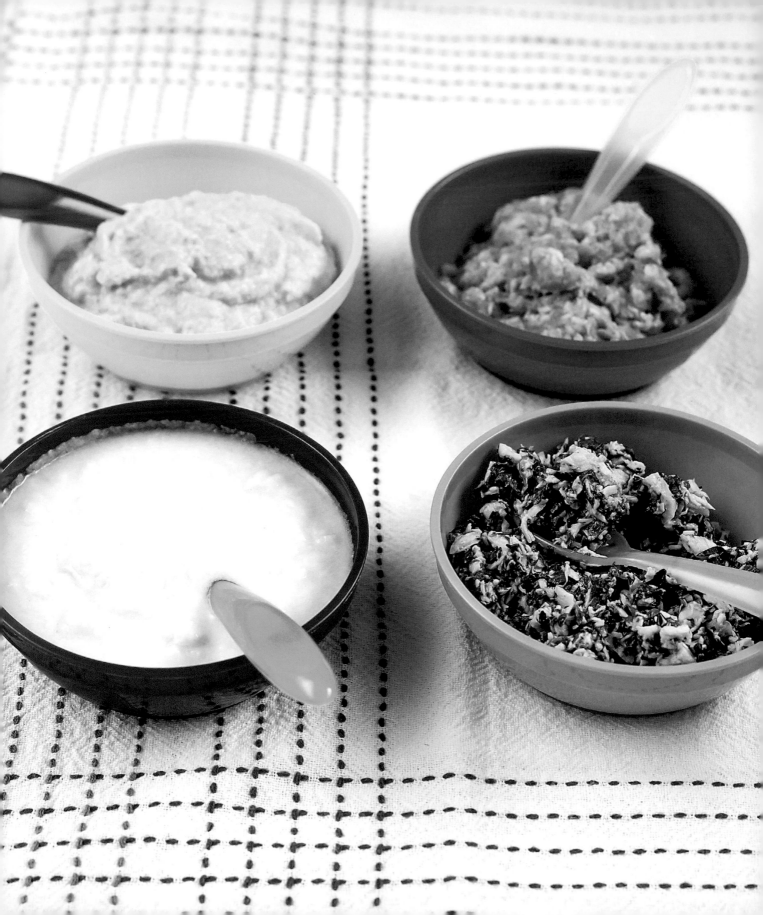

recipes

The recipes in this book allow you to use what you have at home to make delicious homemade baby food. The recipes are broken up by primary food ingredient. For each food there is a step-by-step guide on how to prepare and cook the ingredient, suggestions for tasty mix-ins, and suggestions for when to introduce different foods and textures.

To make life a little easier, there are also adult recipes for each main ingredient designed to feed two hungry parents—and by parents I mean any significant caregiver to baby. This allows you to choose one ingredient, like carrots, and find dinner inspiration for the whole family.

helpful hints

✳ Once you get the basics, come up with your own variations for mix-ins. Just be sure to use ingredients suitable for your baby's age.

✳ Read through the entire recipe before cooking. Sometimes you can cook multiple ingredients together to help save time.

✳ To avoid purees that are too soupy, add just a few tablespoons of liquid at a time until you reach the right consistency.

✳ These recipes were thoroughly tested but the power and efficiency of ovens, stovetops, and microwaves, and the size of fruit, vegetables, and meats may vary. Adjust recipes as necessary.

✳ Play around with flavors by choosing different cooking methods.

✳ You don't need to buy specialty foods to raise a healthy baby. But if there are ingredients that are new to you in this book, I encourage you to try them! You never know—you could find your new favorite food!

nourishing yourself

When you eat well, you feel good. And when your body gets what it needs, you are more likely to feel calm and content and are more capable to handle life's challenges. Long days don't feel as hard. You'll find healthy and nutritious adult recipes in this book with some comforting and indulgent ones mixed in for those days when you need to treat yourself. They are recipes for real life— meals that are ready in 10, 20, and 30 minutes, as well as slow cook meals that you can set and forget. As you nourish your little one, remember to nourish your body. Choose mostly healthy meals, scattered with some indulgent ones for those times when you really need it.

happy tummies

how to make baby food using this book

1. select an ingredient
2. prepare it
3. follow the cooking directions
4. make a simple puree or add mix-ins
5. let cool to room temperature and serve!

recipes yield

* simply baby food recipes generally make 1 cup
* baby food recipes with mix-ins normally make 1½–2½ cups
* 12-month recipes are occasionally single servings
* all adult recipes make 2 servings unless otherwise noted

icon guide

Throughout the book you will see these handy icons. Here's what they mean:

buy organic
Foods with this icon have the highest exposure to pesticides as identified by the Environmental Working Group.[33] Splurge on organic whenever possible.

allergenic foods
Foods that are traditionally known to cause allergies in infants. Check with your doctor before introducing any of these foods if you suspect your baby could be allergic.

grocery store tip
Strategies and techniques for choosing the right products and ingredients at the grocery store.

cook's tip
Useful kitchen tips and tricks.

fruits

apples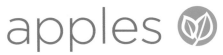

It's true—an apple a day may actually keep the doctor away! Apples are terrific for the body because they are high in vitamin C, fiber, and antioxidants. They also boost energy, lower bad cholesterol, and lessen chances of cardiovascular disease, breast cancer, and osteoporosis.

apple baby food

START WITH 2 apples

1. prep

Wash the apples, then peel and cut into quarters. Remove the core and seeds.

To shorten preparation time, try using an apple peeler, which will core, slice, and peel your apple in just a few seconds!

2. cook

Choose any of these ways to cook your apples.

MICROWAVE

cook time: 3 minutes

Place the apples in a microwave-safe bowl with a splash of water. Microwave on high until tender, about 3–4 minutes.

BOIL

cook time: 8 minutes

Fill half of a medium saucepan with water, and then bring to a boil. Add the apples, then lower the heat to medium low. Cover, and let simmer 8–15 minutes, or until tender. Drain the water.

STEAM

cook time: 12 minutes

Set up a steamer basket in a medium pot and add water so it reaches just below the basket. Bring to a boil. Add the apples, then cover and steam until tender, about 12 minutes.

BAKE

cook time: 15 minutes

Preheat oven to 375°F. Slice the apples, and then place on a sheet pan lined with parchment paper. Bake for 15 minutes or until tender.

3. add mix-ins & serve

Serve simple, or with tasty mix-ins. Puree, roughly mash, or dice according to your baby's stage.

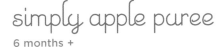

simply apple puree

6 months +

MIX-INS

¼ cup breast milk, formula, or water

....

Puree the apples in a food processor until smooth.

apple oatmeal

7 months +

MIX-INS

½ cup homemade oat infant cereal

2 tablespoons breast milk, formula, or water

Start by bringing 1½ cups of water to a boil in a small saucepan. Reduce heat to low, and then slowly pour the oat infant cereal into the boiling water while stirring with a whisk to prevent clumping. Keep stirring until the cereal is fully mixed into the water, about one minute. Cook for 5 more minutes, until thickened, stirring occasionally. Meanwhile, place the apples in a food processor and puree until smooth. In a small bowl, stir the oat infant cereal, apples, and breast milk, formula, or water together until combined.

apple-plum puree

8 months +

MIX-INS

2 plums

2 tablespoons breast milk, formula, or water

Place whole plums in a saucepan, and cover with water. Bring to a boil and simmer for 2–4 minutes, or until tender. Let cool slightly, then halve, pit, and peel the plums. Place the plums, apples, and breast milk, formula, or water in a food processor and pulse to create a smooth, thick puree.

apple-blueberry puree

9 months +

MIX-INS

½ cup blueberries

2 tablespoons breast milk, formula, or water

Place the apples, blueberries, and breast milk, formula, or water in a food processor and pulse to form a soft, chunky puree.

apple-prune puree

10 months +

MIX-INS

⅓ cup prunes

Bring 1 cup of water to a boil in a small saucepan, then add the prunes. Cook for 5 minutes, or until the prunes are plump, then remove the prunes with a slotted spoon. Place the apples and prunes in a food processor and pulse to create a chunky puree.

pork with apples

11 months +

MIX-INS

1 small boneless pork chop

Cook pork through (bake for 30 minutes at 350°F, broil for 8 minutes, or pan sauté for 8 minutes). Meanwhile, cut the apple into small chunks. Dice the pork into pea-sized cubes, and then mix with apples in a small bowl and serve as finger food or puree until chunky.

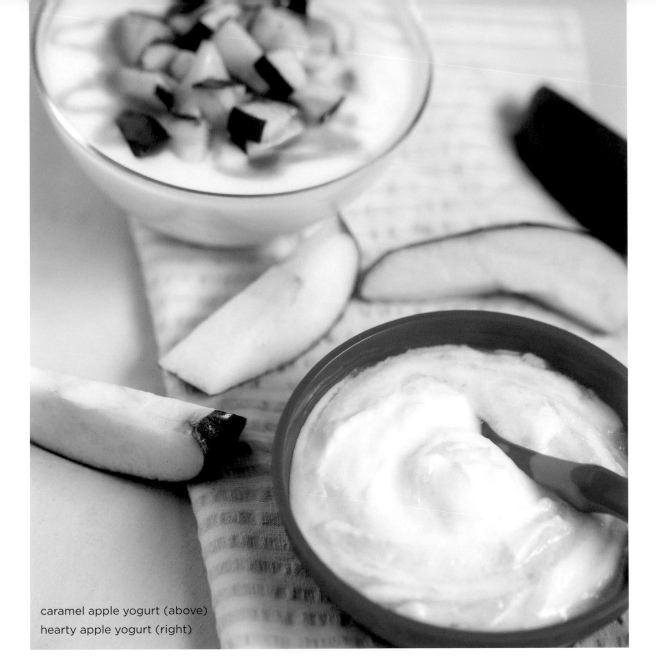

caramel apple yogurt (above)
hearty apple yogurt (right)

hearty apple yogurt

12 months +

MIX-INS

½ **cup plain yogurt**

2 tablespoons wheat germ

Place the apple in a food processor and pulse to make a chunky puree. Stir the apple puree and wheat germ into yogurt until combined.

easy homemade cinnamon applesauce

preparation time: 10 minutes
cook time: 10 minutes

Applesauce is a great midday or after dinner snack. It's light and refreshing, and can tame the fiercest sweet cravings.

6 medium apples

1 cup apple cider with spices (or apple juice, plus 1 teaspoon cinnamon)

Quarter and core the apples. Place the apples and cider in a microwave-safe container and add the lid, lifting one of the corners so steam can escape. Microwave on high for 10 minutes or until soft.

Place the apples and cider in a blender and puree until smooth. Serve warm, or chill in the refrigerator until cold.

turkey apple cheddar wrap

preparation time: 10 minutes

2 tortillas

2 tablespoons honey mustard

⅓ lbs. sliced deli turkey

4 slices cheddar cheese

½ granny smith apple, sliced

1 cup bagged chopped lettuce

Spread each tortilla evenly with honey mustard. Layer turkey, cheese, apple, and lettuce in the center of the tortilla, then roll like a burrito and tuck in the ends. Eat right away or wrap in plastic wrap and keep in the refrigerator, eating within 24 hours.

caramel apple yogurt

preparation time: 5 minutes

2 cups vanilla yogurt

2 large red apples, diced

2 tablespoons caramel sauce

Spoon the yogurt into two bowls or parfait cups. Top with apples and drizzle with caramel sauce.

bananas

Packed with potassium, vitamin B6, vitamin C, and fiber, bananas are extremely nutritious. They're good for your bones, cartilage, and tendons, and help your body heal faster. And there is strong evidence that they can keep your immune system strong, steady your cholesterol, and reduce pre-menstrual and depression symptoms.

banana baby food

START WITH 1 banana

1. prep

Peel banana, and cut off any brown or bruised parts.

2. add mix-ins & serve

Serve simple, or with tasty mix-ins. Puree, roughly mash, or dice according to your baby's stage.

simply banana puree

6 months +

MIX-INS

2 bananas, peeled

1 tablespoon breast milk, formula, or water

Place the bananas and breast milk, formula, or water in a food processor. Puree until smooth and soupy.

banana-pear puree

7 months +

MIX-INS

1 pear

1 tablespoon breast milk, formula, or water

Wash and peel the pear. Cut it in half, and then remove the core and seeds. Cook the pear (microwave for 2 minutes, steam for 3–5 minutes, boil for 10 minutes, or roast for 15 minutes at 425°F). Place the banana, pear, and breast milk, formula, or water in a food processor and puree until smooth.

banana-butternut squash puree

8 months +

MIX-INS

1 cup butternut squash, peeled and cubed

2 tablespoons breast milk, formula, or water

Cook the squash (microwave for 5–15 minutes, boil or steam for 12 minutes, or roast at 400°F for 30 minutes). Place the squash, banana, and breast milk, formula, or water in a food processor and puree to a smooth and thick consistency.

banana-sweet potato mash

9 months +

MIX-INS

1 sweet potato

2 tablespoons water

Wash the potato, and then use a fork to poke holes all over. Place in a microwave-safe dish and microwave for 6–8 minutes, flipping half way through. Cook until tender. Cut in half, and then scoop the inside of the potato into a medium bowl. Mash the banana and sweet potato together to make a soft puree with tiny lumps.

banana oatmeal

10 months +

MIX-INS

½ cup rolled oats

Bring 1 cup of water to a boil in a small saucepan. Lower the heat. Then stir in oats and cook for 5 minutes or until the water is absorbed. Transfer the oatmeal and banana to a food processor and pulse 2–3 times to make a chunky puree.

banana-peach yogurt

11 months +

MIX-INS

½ peach

¼ cup plain Greek yogurt

¼ cup breast milk, formula, or water

Place the banana, peach, yogurt, and breast milk, formula, or water in a food processor. Puree until smooth.

frozen banana puree

12 months +

MIX-INS

1 banana, peeled

⅓ cup breast milk, formula, or water

Wrap one of the bananas in aluminum foil. Freeze for 8 hours or overnight. Place bananas and breast milk, formula, or water in a food processor, and puree until smooth and creamy.

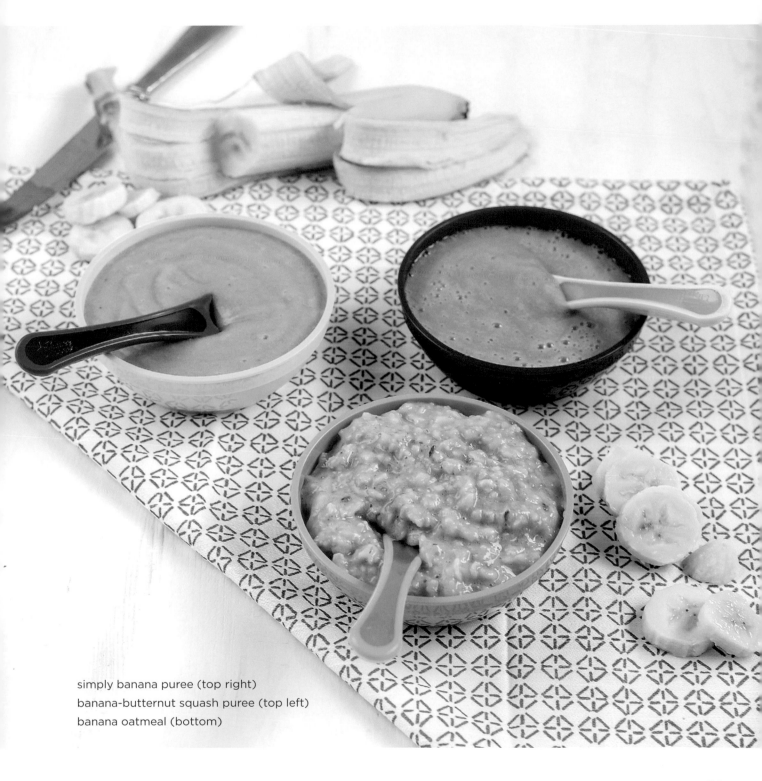

simply banana puree (top right)

banana-butternut squash puree (top left)

banana oatmeal (bottom)

bananas

maple walnut banana porridge

preparation time: 5 minutes

cook time: 7 minutes

This is my all-time favorite hot cereal recipe. It's warm, comforting, and filling—perfect for those chilly mornings.

½ **cup quick steel cut oats**

1 **banana, sliced**

¼ **cup milk**

½ **teaspoon cinnamon**

¼ **cup walnuts**

2 **tablespoons real maple syrup**

Bring 1¼ cups of water to a boil in a medium saucepan.

Stir in the oatmeal and banana slices, then reduce heat and simmer for 5–7 minutes. Stir on occasion to keep the oatmeal from sticking to the bottom.

Turn the burner off and stir in the milk and cinnamon. Divide between two serving bowls, and top with walnuts and maple syrup. Serve piping hot.

skinny monkey ice cream

preparation time: overnight freezing + 5 minutes

2 **bananas**

½ **cup milk**

2 **tablespoon confectioner's sugar**

⅓ **cup dark chocolate chips**

⅓ **cup walnuts**

Peel the bananas, and then wrap them in aluminum foil and freeze overnight.

Cut the bananas in half, and place them in a blender with the milk and sugar. Whirl on high until smooth. Scoop the banana ice cream into 2 serving bowls. Top with chocolate chips and walnuts.

peanut butter banana pancakes

preparation time: 5 minutes

cook time: 15 minutes

1 **cup just-add-water pancake mix**

¼ **cup peanut butter**

1 **tablespoon butter**

2 **bananas, peeled and cut into ¼-inch wheels**

Whisk the pancake mix, peanut butter, and ¾ cup water together in a medium bowl until combined.

Heat a nonstick skillet over medium heat and melt enough butter to lightly coat the pan. Pour batter onto the skillet, using about ¼ of the batter to make a medium-sized pancake.

Scatter the pancake with banana slices, pushing them into the batter. Flip when the top of the pancake is bubbly. Cook until golden brown and cooked through. Remove the pancake and place on a serving plate.

Use a paper towel to carefully wipe and clean the skillet, and then place the pan back on the burner. Add the remaining butter and repeat instructions for the rest of the pancake batter. Serve piping hot. No syrup needed.

chocolate hazelnut banana toast

4 slices whole wheat bread

⅛ cup chocolate hazelnut spread

½ banana, sliced

Toast the bread, and then smear a thin layer of chocolate hazelnut spread on top. Top it off with banana slices.

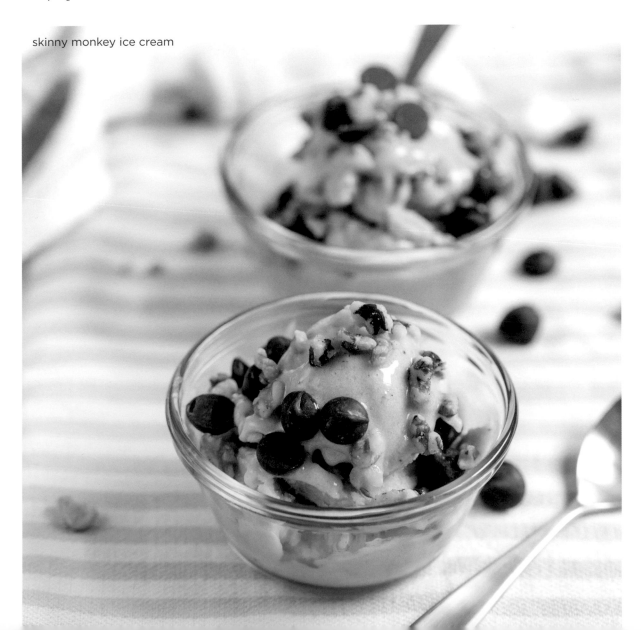

skinny monkey ice cream

blueberries

These little berries have tremendous health benefits. To start, they are an excellent source of antioxidants, copper, vitamin K, and fiber. A diet rich in these nutrients helps promote healthy skin, eyes, heart, urinary tract, immune system, memory, and cholesterol. Blueberries are also a natural anti-inflammatory, and help reduce the risk of certain cancers.

 Fresh blueberries don't need to be cooked for babies. Just pick through, wash, and puree.

blueberry baby food

START WITH 3 cups of fresh blueberries

1. prep

Look over the blueberries, and pick out overripe or deteriorated berries. Remove any stems. Thoroughly clean by washing well under cool water, or make a vinegar bath by placing the blueberries in a bowl and adding 1½ cups of cool water and 1½ cups of white vinegar. Let the blueberries soak for 2 minutes. Then pour them into a colander and drain the water. Rinse well.

2. add mix-ins & serve

Serve simple or with tasty mix-ins. Puree, roughly mash, or cut in half according to your baby's stage.

simply blueberry puree
8 months +

Place the blueberries in a blender and puree until smooth and thick. Strain the puree in a fine mesh strainer to remove the seeds if desired.

blueberry-pear puree
9 months +

MIX-INS
1 pear

Peel the pear, and then cut it into quarters and remove the core and seeds. Cook the pear until tender (microwave for 2 minutes, steam for 3–5 minutes, boil for 10 minutes, or roast for 15 minutes at 425°). Place the blueberries and pear in a blender. Blitz to form a coarse and chunky puree.

blueberry-banana puree

10 months +

MIX-INS

1 banana, peeled

Transfer the blueberries and banana to a blender and pulse to a fine dice.

pork with blueberries

11 months +

MIX-INS

1 pork chop

Heat a skillet over medium heat. Add ½ table-spoon of oil, and then add the pork chop. Cook for 2 minutes to brown the pork chop, then flip and add ⅓ cup blueberries. (Reserve the rest of the blueberries for another meal or a snack.) Continue cooking until the pork chop is cooked through. Pulse the blueberries and pork chop together to form a coarse and chunky puree, or finely dice the pork and mix with the blueberries to serve as finger food.

blueberry cottage cheese

12 months +

MIX-INS

½ cup full-fat cottage cheese

½ cup blueberries

Thoroughly mash or puree the blueberries until smooth. Spoon a serving of cottage cheese into a baby food bowl, and then swirl in 2–3 tablespoons of blueberry puree.

blueberry yogurt smoothie

total time: 5 minutes

½ cup low-fat milk

1 ripe banana

1 cup blueberries

½ cup Greek vanilla yogurt

1 tablespoon ground flax seeds

½ cup ice

Place the blueberries and banana in a blender and pulse to finely dice.

pork tenderloin with blueberry sauce

total time: 10 minutes

1 tablespoon canola oil

2 pork chops

½ teaspoon dried thyme

¾ cup blueberries

1 tablespoon butter

Heat the oil in a medium skillet, then add the pork chops. Brown one side, then flip.

Sprinkle the pork with thyme, and then add the blueberries and butter. Cook until the pork is cooked through, about 8 minutes total.

blueberry crepes with vanilla yogurt

total time: 5 minutes

2 store-bought crepes

1 cup blueberries

confectioner's sugar, optional

Greek or whole milk vanilla yogurt

Heat the crepes in the microwave for 5–10 seconds, or until warm. Place the blueberries in the center of the crepes, then fold the sides over to completely cover the filling. Sprinkle with powdered sugar, if desired, then top each with a dollop of yogurt.

figs

Figs offer an excellent source of fiber, potassium, copper, vitamin B6, and calcium. These nutrients help you feel full longer, and are important for metabolism and immunity. They also help aid in digestion, and help babies build strong bones.

For women, figs are a great snack during that treacherous time of the month. They reduce bloating and moodiness prior to menstruation. Unlike most dried fruits, dried figs contain more nutrients than fresh ones.

Though hard to find, fresh figs make a fast meal for baby because they don't need to be cooked before being served. They are soft and have a mild, sweet flavor.

fig baby food

START WITH 6 fresh figs or 1 cup of dried figs

1. prep

Wash the fresh figs. Then remove the stems and cut in half. Dried figs are ready as is.

2. cook

Fresh figs don't need to be cooked. Plump dried figs before serving.

PLUMPING DRIED FIGS

cook time: 5 minutes

Place the dried figs in a small bowl and cover them with boiling water. Let sit for 5–10 minutes or until plump and soft. Slice off the stems. Some of the nutrients may leak out of the figs and into the water, so save some of the cooking water to help thin out baby's purees and retain the lost nutrients.

3. add mix-ins & serve

Serve simple, or with tasty mix-ins. Puree or dice according to your baby's stage.

simply fig puree
7 months +

MIX-INS

2 tablespoons breast milk, formula, or water for fresh figs (1¼ cups for dried figs)

Place figs, breast milk, formula, or water in a blender and puree until smooth. The mixture should have a soupy consistency. Strain the seeds using a fine mesh sieve if desired.

figgy pear puree

8 months +

MIX-INS

1 pear

Peel, quarter, and core one pear. Cook until tender (microwave for 2 minutes, steam for 3–5 minutes, boil for 10 minutes, or roast for 15 minutes at 425°F). Carefully transfer the pear to a food processor with the figs and puree until smooth.

figs and cottage cheese

9 months +

MIX-INS

½ cup whole milk cottage cheese

1 cup breast milk, formula, or cooking water (if using dried figs)

Puree the fresh figs by themselves, or the dried figs with the breast milk, formula, or cooking water in a food processor until smooth. Place the cottage cheese in a bowl and mash to create tiny, soft lumps. Swirl in 2–3 tablespoons of fig puree, reserving the remaining fig puree for another meal.

fig-apricot puree

10 months +

MIX-INS

2 fresh apricots (or 1 cup of dried apricots)

1 cup breast milk, formula, or cooking water (if using dried fruit)

If using fresh apricots, halve them, slicing around the pit, and then remove the stone. Cook until soft and tender (microwave for 2 minutes, steam for 5 minutes, or roast at 400°F for 15 minutes). If using dried apricots, place them in a bowl and cover with hot water. Then let them sit until plump and soft. Puree the figs and apricots (with the cooking water if using dried fruit) to create a chunky puree.

yogurt and figs

11 months +

MIX-INS

1¼ cups yogurt

1¼ cups breast milk, formula, or cooking water (if using dried figs)

Puree the fresh figs by themselves, or the dried figs with the breast milk, formula, or cooking water in a food processor until smooth. You can strain the seeds if you prefer the dish completely smooth. Place ½ cup of yogurt in a bowl and swirl in 2–3 tablespoons of fig puree, reserving the remaining yogurt and fig puree for another meal.

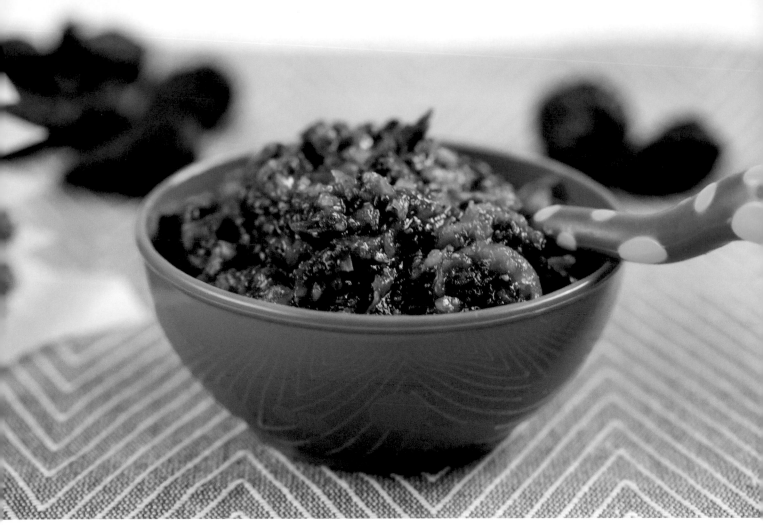

fig-apricot puree

figgy oats
12 months +

MIX-INS

½ cup rolled oats

1 cup breast milk, formula, or cooking water
(if using dried figs)

1 tablespoon breast milk or formula

Bring 2 cups of water to a boil in a medium sauce-pan. Add oats, and then simmer for 5 minutes. Meanwhile, puree the figs in a food processor, adding a cup of breast milk, formula, or water if using dried figs. Stir the fig puree and remaining tablespoon of liquid into the oats to make a creamy, sweet oatmeal.

strawberry-fig spinach salad

total time: 10 minutes

2 cups fresh spinach

¾ cup sliced strawberries

⅓ cup dried figs, or 4 fresh figs, diced

2 tablespoons sliced almonds

balsamic dressing

Wash the spinach, and then blot with a paper towel or use a salad spinner to dry the leaves.

Divide the spinach between two serving bowls. Top with the strawberries, figs, sliced almonds, and balsamic dressing.

fig-almond oatmeal

total time: 10 minutes

⅓ cup diced dried figs

1 cup cooked oatmeal

1 tablespoon sliced almonds

Place figs in a hot water bath for 5 minutes until plump. Remove the stems, and then place in a food processor with a splash of hot water. Finely dice figs.

Meanwhile, prepare oatmeal just how you like it. Stir figs into the steaming hot bowl of oatmeal. Top with almonds.

no-bake coconut fig bars

total time: 15 minutes

These irresistible no-bake snack bars are packed with energy boosting nutrients, so they'll keep you going between meals.

1 cup dried figs, stemmed

¾ cup dried apricots

1 cup whole raw almonds

½ cup sweetened shredded coconut

1 tablespoon chia seeds

2 tablespoons coconut oil

Place all of the ingredients in a food processor and pulse to form a sticky dough.

Line an 8 × 8 square baking dish with parchment paper, and then pour in the dough. Press the dough into the bottom of the dish to create an even layer.

Refrigerate for 20 minutes to firm, and then slice into bars. Wrap each bar with plastic wrap for easy grab-and-go snacks, or wrap the whole baking dish. Store in the refrigerator.

no-bake coconut fig bars

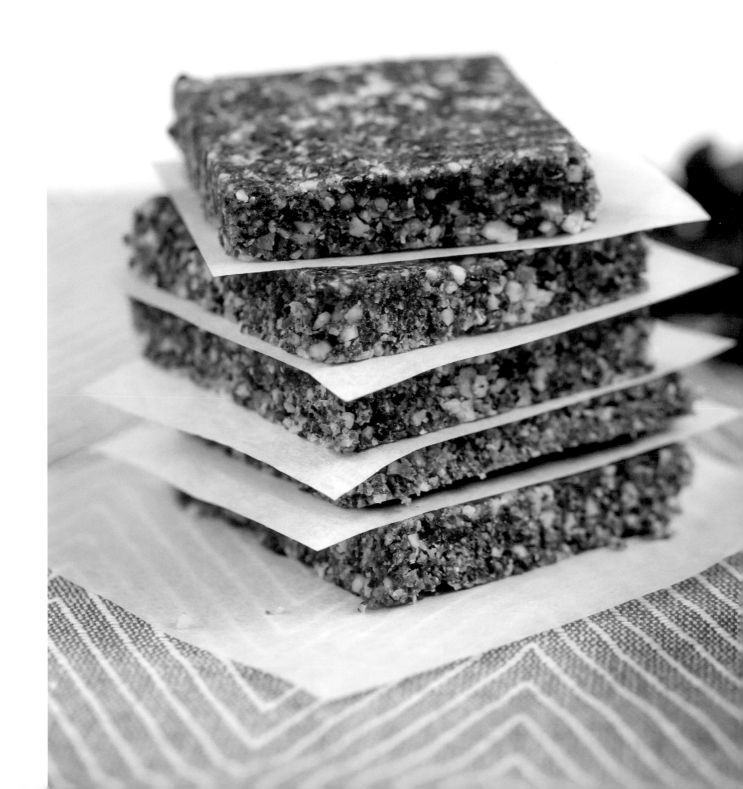

kiwifruits

Kiwifruit is an excellent source of vitamins C, E, and K, fiber, and potassium, promoting healthy vision, digestion, and immunity. It is also great for cardio-vascular health, preventing clogged arteries and lowering bad blood pressure.

The tiny black seeds inside kiwifruit are edible, but if you'd like to remove them for baby, just press the fruit through a fine mesh strainer.

kiwifruit baby food

START WITH 1 kiwifruit

1. prep

Cut off the ends of the kiwifruit, and then stand it up on one side. Using a paring knife, carefully slice off the skin. Then chop the fruit.

2. add mix-ins and serve

Serve on its own, or with tasty mix-ins. Puree, mash, or dice according to your baby's stage.

kiwi-banana puree

8 months +

MIX-INS

¾ banana, peeled

1 tablespoon breast milk, formula, or water

Place the peeled banana, chopped kiwifruit, and breast milk, formula, or water in a food processor. Puree until smooth and thick.

Kiwifruit allergies are increasingly common in children, especially when someone in baby's family has a citrus or latex allergy. Check with your doctor if you suspect your baby may have a problem with this ingredient.

Since kiwifruit can be acidic, you might want to pair it with a mild ingredient that your baby is familiar with (like bananas) before feeding it to him on its own.

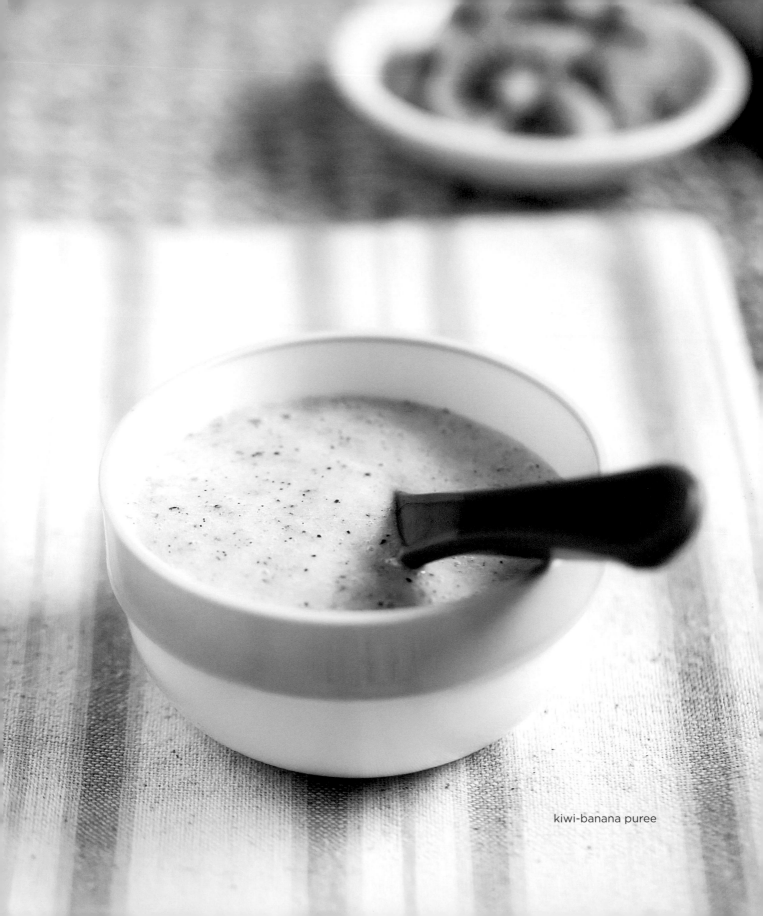

kiwi-banana puree

kiwi, apple, and banana puree

9 months +

MIX-INS

1 apple

1 banana, peeled

1 tablespoon breast milk, formula, or water

Peel the apple, and then cut it in half and remove the core and seeds. Cook the apple until tender (microwave for 4 minutes, boil for 10 minutes, steam for 12 minutes, or bake for 15 minutes at 375°F). Let cool slightly. Place the apple, banana, kiwifruit, and breast milk, formula, or water in a food processor and puree to form a soft, lumpy puree.

kiwi, pear, and spinach puree

10 months +

MIX-INS

1 pear

1 cup fresh spinach, washed

Peel the pear, and then quarter and remove the core and seeds. Place the pear and spinach in a microwave-safe dish with 1 tablespoon of water and cook for 2–3 minutes, or until tender. Let cool slightly. Place the kiwifruit, pear, and spinach in a blender. Blitz to make a chunky puree.

kiwi-blueberry yogurt smoothie

11 months +

MIX-INS

1½ cups blueberries

⅓ cup Greek yogurt

⅓ cup breast milk, formula, or water

Place all of the ingredients in a blender, and puree until smooth.

kiwi-mango salmon

12 months +

MIX-INS

1 small skinless salmon fillet, deboned

⅓ cup diced mango

Meant to be paired with the adult recipe that follows. Place the fish on a hot, oiled grill and cook through, about 7 minutes. Meanwhile, finely dice the kiwifruit and mango. Flake the fish, then place in a small bowl with the fruit. Serve as finger food.

make-ahead fruit and yogurt parfait

preparation time: 10 minutes

This rainbow parfait is made with a variety of fruits, so you get an assortment of colors, flavors, and nutrients. For an easy morning, assemble the parfaits the night before so it's all set for breakfast. You can even double the recipe so you have breakfast ready for the next day too.

1 kiwifruit

½ orange, or 1 clementine

5 strawberries

¼ cup blueberries

¼ cup walnuts

3 cups nonfat plain Greek yogurt

Peel the kiwifruit and orange, and then dice. Slice the strawberries.

In a tall glass, plastic container, or mason jar, layer the yogurt, fruit, and walnuts. Cover and refrigerate until morning.

salmon with kiwi-mango salsa

preparation time: 10 minutes

cook time: 8 minutes

2 (6-ounce) salmon fillets

2 tablespoons olive oil

2 kiwifruits, diced

½ cup mango, diced

2 tablespoons cilantro, roughly chopped

Preheat the grill or grill pan to medium heat.

Brush both sides of the fish with olive oil, and season with salt and pepper. Peel and dice the mango and kiwifruit and place in a small bowl. Stir in the cilantro. Refrigerator to chill until serving time.

Grill the fish for 5–7 minutes, or until it flakes with a fork. Place onto serving plates and top with salsa.

kiwi banana breakfast granola

preparation time: 5 minutes

1 cup granola

1 kiwifruit, peeled and chopped

2 bananas, sliced

1 cup milk

Divide granola into two bowls. Top each with kiwifruit and bananas, then pour on the milk.

mangoes

Mango is a sweet tropical fruit that is low in calories and high in vitamin A. It is also a good source of vitamins C, E, and K, potassium, and copper. These nutrients are excellent for new mothers because they promote faster healing from wounds and bruising, protect the body from infection, and regulate mood, sleep, and stress.

Ripe mangoes are slightly soft and have a fragrant smell.

mango baby food

START WITH 2 mangoes or 1½ cups frozen mango cubes

1. prep

Wash the mangoes, and then remove the pit in the center of the fruit. To do so, stand the mango up on one side. Using a paring knife, carefully cut the mango in half, just to the right of the center. If you hit the pit, move your knife over slightly so it moves through the mango easily. Make another slice down the other side, and then throw out the pit. Next, remove the peel from the fruit by slicing a checkerboard pattern into the mango. Try to keep the knife from going through the skin. Flip the skin so that the mango pieces stick out, and then carefully cut off the mango cubes.

Slicing mango can be tricky if you haven't done it before, but thanks to the Internet there are lots of videos that show you just how to do it.

If using frozen mango, thaw.

Mangoes do not need to be cooked, but if your baby has a hard time digesting citrus fruits, steam until tender and let cool before pureeing.

2. add mix-ins & serve

Serve on its own, or with tasty mix-ins. Puree or dice according to your baby's stage.

simply mango puree

8 months +

MIX-INS

2 tablespoons breast milk, formula, or water

Place the mango and breast milk, formula, or water in a food processor, and puree until smooth and thick.

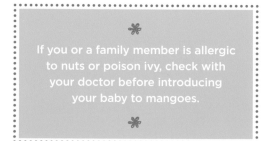

If you or a family member is allergic to nuts or poison ivy, check with your doctor before introducing your baby to mangoes.

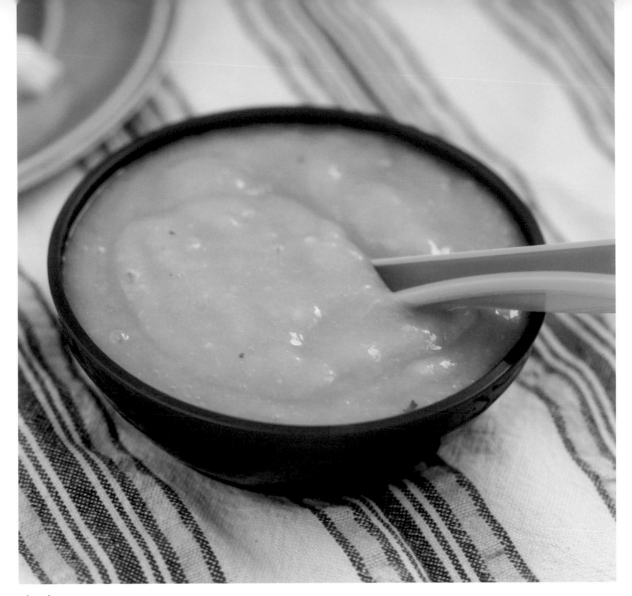

simply mango puree

mango-blueberry puree

9 months +

MIX-INS

½ cup blueberries

....

Place the mango and blueberries in a food processor and pulse to create a coarse and chunky puree.

mango-cantaloupe puree

10 months +

MIX-INS

1 cup cantaloupe, chopped

....

Place the mango and cantaloupe in a food processor and puree until coarse and chunky.

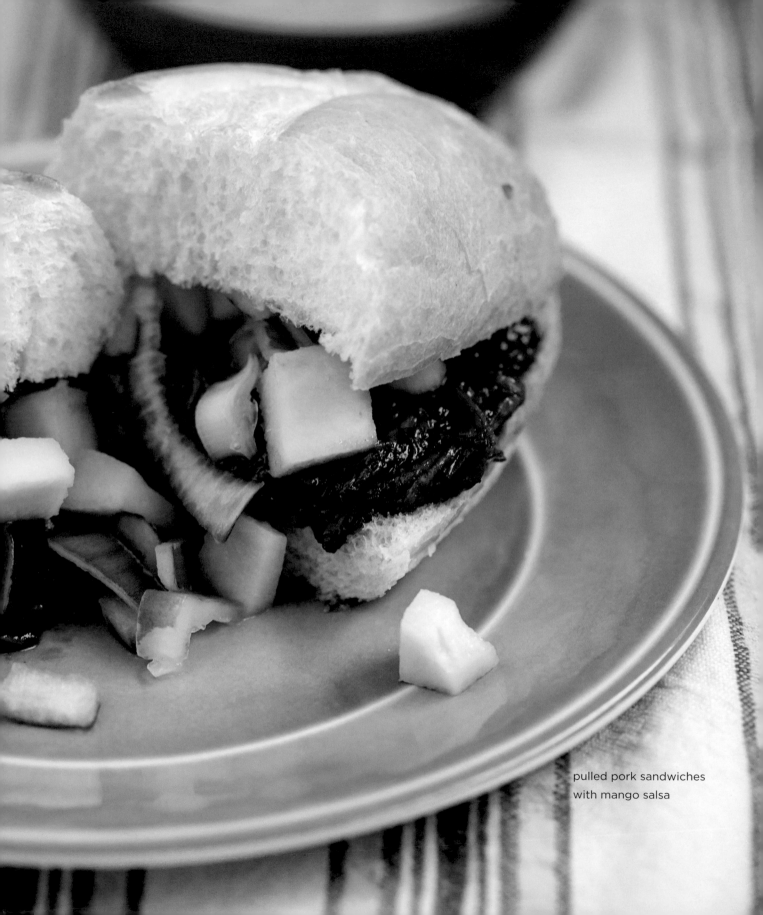

pulled pork sandwiches
with mango salsa

mango-peach oatmeal

11 months +

MIX-INS

¾ cup rolled oats

1 peach, peeled and chopped

1 tablespoon breast milk or formula

Bring 1½ cups of water to a boil in a medium saucepan. Add oats and chopped peaches, and then simmer for 5 minutes. Drain any excess water from the oatmeal, and then place the mango, oats, peaches, and breast milk or formula in a food processor and puree until coarse and chunky.

mango chicken

12 months +

MIX-INS

⅓ cup diced chicken

Cook chicken until no longer pink (poach for 10 minutes, grill for 6–10 minutes per side, sauté for 10 minutes, or bake for 15 minutes at 375°F). Finely dice the mango and chicken, and then serve a few pieces at a time as finger food.

mama recipes

pulled pork sandwiches with mango salsa

preparation time: 25 minutes

slow-cook time: 8 hours

leftovers: 1–2 meals

1 2-lb. pork shoulder or pork butt

1 (19-ounce) jar brown sugar barbecue sauce

1 mango, peeled and diced

⅓ cup red onion, sliced

spritz of lime juice

soft buns for serving

Spray a slow cooker with cooking spray, and then add the pork and barbecue sauce. Cover and cook on low for 8 hours.

When the pork has about 10 minutes left, toss the mango, onion, and lime juice together in a small bowl.

When the pork is finished cooking, use 2 forks to pull it into shreds. Place a mound of pulled pork on the bottom of two buns, and then top with mango salsa. Serve as open-faced or hand-held sandwiches.

mango-acai bowl

total time: 5 minutes

1 cup chopped mango

1 cup frozen blueberries

1 packet frozen acai berry puree

1 banana

½ cup milk

granola

Add all of the ingredients except for the granola in a blender until smooth, and then pour into a bowl and top with granola.

chicken kabobs with bacon and mango

preparation time: 10 minutes

cook time: 15 minutes

2 chicken breasts

5 slices bacon, cut into 2-inch pieces

1 mango, chopped

½ green or red pepper, chopped

2 tablespoons vegetable oil

metal skewers

Preheat the grill or grill pan to medium heat.

Meanwhile, chop the chicken into 1½ inch cubes. Wrap each piece of chicken with a piece of bacon.

Thread a piece of chicken on the skewer so the bacon is secured. Fill each skewer, alternating with chicken, mango, and peppers. Be careful not to pack too tightly, otherwise the chicken won't cook through. Season with salt and pepper.

Lightly oil the grill grate and place the skewers on the grill. Cook for 10–15 minutes, or until the bacon is crisp and the chicken is cooked through.

coconut-mango curry with shrimp

preparation time: 10 minutes

cook time: 15 minutes

1 mango, peeled and sliced

1 10 oz. can of coconut milk

4 teaspoons spicy curry paste

½ medium yellow onion, chopped

1 cup red pepper, chopped

1 tablespoon vegetable oil

1½ lbs. shrimp, shelled and deveined

To make the coconut mango sauce, place the coconut milk and half of the mango slices in a blender and puree until smooth. Set aside.

Heat a large skillet over medium-high heat and add the oil. Add the curry paste and cook until fragrant, about 1 minute. Add the onion and peppers to the pan and cook until soft, about 5 minutes.

Add the coconut mango sauce and shrimp to the pan. Cook until the shrimp turn pink and the sauce is hot. Serve the curry with rice and fresh mango on the side.

melons

Honeydew and cantaloupe melons are packed with potassium, vitamins A, C, and B6, fiber, and folate. These nutrients help boost mood, and regulate stress and sleep. They are great for your immune system, eyes, and heart, and also keep you hydrated.

melon baby food

START WITH 2 cups cubed honeydew or cantaloupe melon

1. prep

Cut a melon in half, and then scoop out the seeds. Cover half the melon with plastic wrap and place it in the refrigerator. Peel and chop the other half.

Melon does not need to be cooked, but if you want to make it easier to digest, steam until tender and let cool before pureeing.

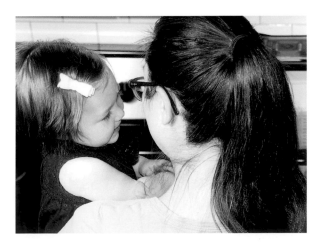

2. add mix-ins & serve

Serve on its own or with tasty mix-ins. Experiment with temperature, using frozen ingredients mixed with melon to make cool treats.

simply melon puree
9 months +

Place the melon in a blender and puree until mostly smooth with tiny lumps.

cantaloupe-banana puree
10 months +

MIX-INS
1 banana

Mash the cantaloupe and banana together to make a soft, slightly lumpy puree.

cantaloupe-peach yogurt

11 months +

MIX-INS

1 peach

½ cup yogurt

Cut the peach in half, and then remove the pit. Cook the peach until tender (2 minutes in the microwave, 5 minutes steamed, or 8–10 minutes boiled). When the peach is cool, peel off the skin. Place the fruit and yogurt in a blender and puree until smooth.

cool strawberry-cantaloupe puree

12 months +

MIX-INS

1½ cups frozen strawberries

Puree the melon and strawberries together until smooth.

mama recipes

strawberry-cantaloupe sorbet

preparation time: 5 minutes

freezer time: 3 hours

leftovers: 2 servings

3 cups frozen, chopped cantaloupe

2 cups frozen strawberries

½ cup orange juice

¾ cup water

Place the frozen cantaloupe, strawberries, orange juice, and water in a blender and puree until smooth. Scoop into serving bowls. Store any remaining sorbet in the freezer in a freezer-safe container.

melon-peach smoothie

preparation time: 5 minutes

3 cups cantaloupe, chopped

1 peach, halved and pitted

½ cup plain Greek yogurt

Place the cantaloupe, peach, and yogurt in a blender and puree until smooth. Pour into serving glasses and serve.

papayas

Papaya is an excellent source of potassium, fiber, folate, and vitamins C, A, and E. Papaya eases pain and reduces inflammation in the body, and some research suggests that it may protect against some illnesses, like cancer.

The seeds of the papaya are edible and have many health benefits, such as killing parasites in the intestinal system. So if you have an upset stomach, you may want to throw some papaya seeds into a smoothie or a salad for relief.

 You can tell that a papaya is ripe if it is yellow or golden in color, and gives a little when you touch it.

papaya baby food

START WITH 1 cup papaya

1. prep

Wash a fully ripened papaya and cut in half. Using a large spoon, remove the seeds and save them in a plastic bag if you plan to eat them later on. Scoop out a cup of papaya. Cover and refrigerate any leftover fruit and seeds.

2. add mix-ins and serve

Serve simple, or with tasty mix-ins. Puree, mash, or dice according to your baby's stage.

simply papaya puree
9 months +

Mash papaya with a fork or puree in a food processor to form a soft puree with tiny lumps.

papaya-banana puree
10 months +

MIX-INS
½ **banana, peeled**

Mash the banana and papaya together to combine and form a soft, lumpy puree.

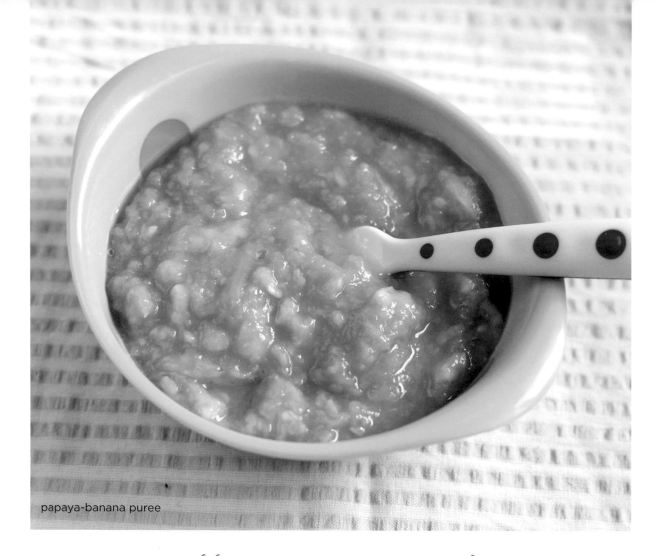

papaya-banana puree

papaya rice pudding

11 months +

MIX-INS
2 tablespoons cooked rice

Mash the papaya until smooth and slightly lumpy. Stir in the rice until combined.

papaya and avocado salad

12 months +

MIX-INS
½ large avocado, pitted

Scoop the avocado flesh out of the skin. Dice the papaya and avocado, and then place in a small bowl and gently toss together. Serve as finger food.

fruits

honey yogurt with papaya

preparation time: 5 minutes

2 cups plain yogurt

2 tablespoons honey

½ cup papaya, diced

¼ cup papaya seeds

Scoop out the seeds from the papaya, and then rinse them under water.

Spoon the yogurt into two bowls and swirl with honey. Top with diced papaya and seeds.

sriracha shrimp with avocado papaya salad

preparation time: 10 minutes

cook time: 5 minutes

2 tablespoons sriracha (Thai hot sauce) or hot sauce of choice

⅓ cup + 1 tablespoon olive oil

1 teaspoon paprika

1½ lbs. medium shrimp, peeled and deveined

½ cup papaya, diced

½ cup avocado, diced

2 tablespoons lemon juice

skewers

Heat the grill to 350°F or a grill pan to medium.

In a medium bowl, whisk together the hot sauce, olive oil, and paprika. Add the shrimp and toss to coat. Cover and place in the refrigerator.

In a small bowl, gently stir together the diced papaya, avocado, and lime juice, and then set aside.

Thread the shrimp on the skewers and cook on the grill for 2–3 minutes per side, or until pink and opaque. Serve shrimp with the avocado papaya salad.

coconut-papaya rice

preparation time: 5 minutes

cook time: 15 minutes

leftovers: 2 servings

This sweet and sticky rice is full of flavor. Serve it with grilled chicken or fish, curry or stir-fry, or warm as dessert.

1 cup coconut milk

¾ cup jasmine rice

1 cup papaya, diced

Bring coconut milk and 1¾ cups of water to a boil over medium-high heat. Add the rice, then cover and simmer for 15 minutes or until tender.

Meanwhile, mash ½ cup of papaya with a fork. Stir the papaya puree into the rice. Scoop the rice into serving bowls and top with remaining papaya.

peaches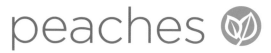

Peaches are a good source of fiber, copper, vitamins C and E, and niacin. A diet rich in these nutrients helps to keep your eyes, heart, and immune systems healthy. They may also prevent tumors and cancerous cells from growing, and help you maintain healthy blood sugar levels.

peach baby food

START WITH 3 peaches or 2¼ cups frozen, sliced peaches

1. prep

Cut into the peach near the stem, and then run the knife all the way around the fruit, ending where you started. Twist each peach half in opposite directions so that one half comes free from the pit. Use a spoon or knife to remove the pit.

If using frozen peaches, thaw.

2. cook

There are several ways to cook peaches.

MICROWAVE

cook time: 2 minutes

Place peach halves and a splash of water in a microwave-safe bowl. Microwave until the peaches are tender, about 2 minutes. Once the peaches are cool to the touch, remove the peel and slice.

STEAM

cook time: 3 minutes

Set up a steamer basket in a medium pot and add enough water so it reaches just below the basket. Bring to a boil. Cover and steam the peaches until tender, 3–5 minutes. When the peaches are cool to the touch, remove the peel and slice.

ROAST

cook time: 20 minutes

Preheat oven to 425°F. Place the peaches cut side up on a baking dish sprayed with cooking spray. Roast for 20 minutes or until tender. When the peaches are cool to the touch, remove the peel and slice.

3. add mix-ins & serve

simply peach puree

7 months +

Transfer peaches and breast milk, formula, or water to a food processor and puree until smooth.

peach-blueberry puree

8 months +

MIX-INS

½ cup blueberries

Puree the peaches and blueberries in a food processor to create a smooth and thick puree.

peach-tofu puree

9 months +

MIX-INS

¼ cup tofu

Place the peaches and tofu in a food processor and puree to form a thick puree with tiny lumps.

peach-plum puree

10 months +

MIX-INS

3 plums

1 banana, peeled

Peel the plums, then cut in half and remove the pit. Place the plums, peaches, and banana in a food processor and pulse to create a chunky puree.

peach applesauce

11 months +

MIX-INS

1 apple

Peel and chop the apple. Remove the core and seeds. Cook the apple until tender (about 2–3 minutes in the microwave or boil for 10–15 minutes on the stovetop). Pulse the peach and apple in a blender to make a chunky puree.

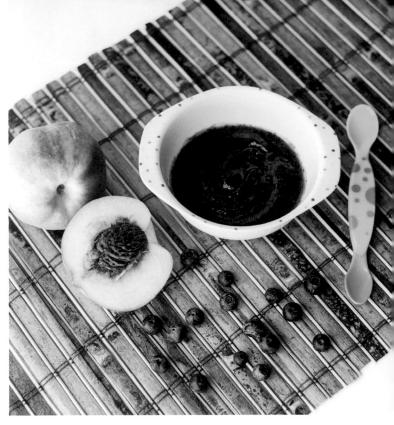

peach-blueberry puree

peaches and cream oatmeal

12 months +

MIX-INS

½ cup rolled oats

2 tablespoons breast milk or formula

Bring 1½ cups of water to a boil in a medium saucepan. Add oats and simmer for 5 minutes. Drain any excess water from the oatmeal, then place the oats, peaches, and breast milk or formula in a food processor and puree until coarse and chunky.

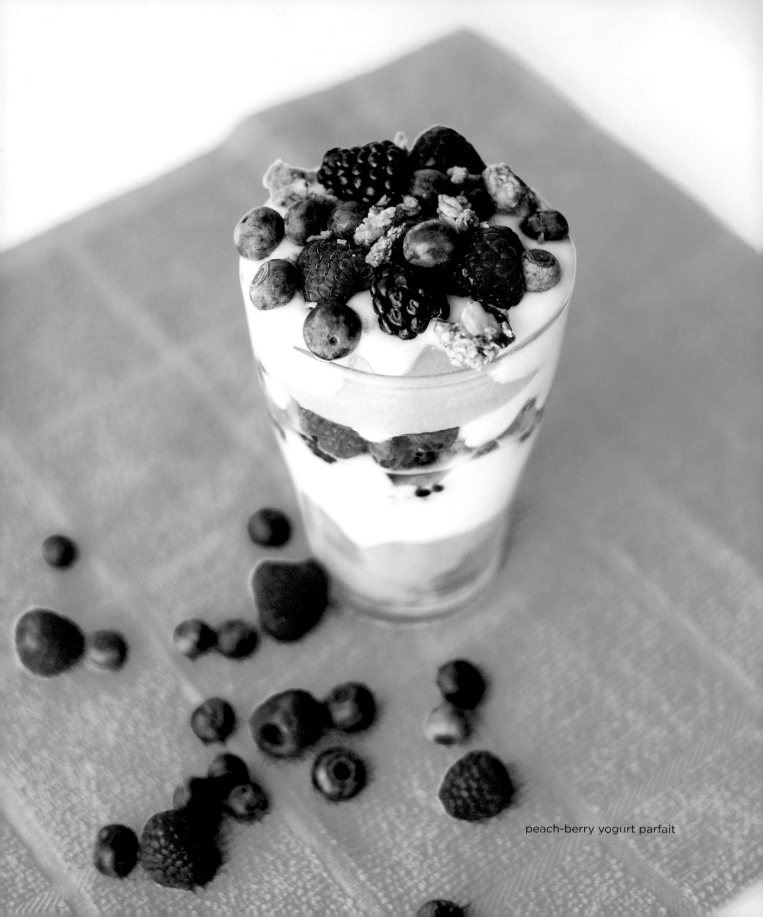

peach-berry yogurt parfait

peach-berry yogurt parfait

preparation time: 5 minutes

When I was in college I used to have this parfait in between classes to boost my energy and regain my focus. As a new mom, I've found it to be a satisfying light breakfast or afternoon snack to refuel me for a day of mothering.

2 cups vanilla yogurt

½ cup mixed berries

1 peach, pitted and sliced

½ cup granola

In two bowls or glasses, layer the yogurt, fruit, and granola. Cover and refrigerate or serve immediately.

baked french toast with peaches

preparation time: 10 minutes

cook time: 10 minutes

4 eggs

⅛ cup milk

2 tablespoons confectioner's sugar

⅛ teaspoon cinnamon

1 teaspoon vanilla

5 pieces of white bread

1 peach, sliced

maple syrup, for serving

Heat oven to 400°F. Line a baking sheet with parchment paper.

Crack the eggs in a bowl and whisk until smooth. Whisk in milk, confectioner's sugar, cinnamon, and vanilla. One at a time, dunk the bread slices into the egg mixture, letting the extra egg drip off. Place the bread on the baking sheet, and add the peach slices wherever there is room.

Bake for 7 minutes, and then flip the toast. It should be golden brown on the bottom. Continue cooking until both sides of the toast are browned.

Serve the French toast with sliced peaches and a drizzle of maple syrup.

pears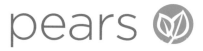

Pears are high in fiber, copper, and vitamins C and K. These nutrients promote a healthy urinary tract, immune system, memory, and heart. They may also fight wrinkles, promote good vision, and reduce the risk of certain cancers.

pear baby food

START WITH 1 pear

1. prep

Wash and peel the pear. Quarter, and then remove the core and seeds.

2. cook

There are several ways to cook pears.

MICROWAVE

cook time: 2 minutes

Place the pear and 1 teaspoon of water in a microwave-safe bowl. Cover, leaving a small space to let the steam out. Cook on high for 2 minutes, or until the pear is soft.

STEAM

cook time: 3 minutes

Set up a steamer basket in a medium pot. Add enough water so it reaches just below the basket. Bring to a boil, and then add the pears to the basket. Cover and steam for 3-5 minutes or until the pears are tender.

SAUTÉ

cook time: 6 minutes

Chop the pears. Heat a nonstick skillet over medium heat, and then add ½ tablespoon of butter. Add the pears. Stir often until the pears are tender, about 6–8 minutes.

ROAST

cook time: 15 minutes

Preheat oven to 425°F. Place the pears on a baking sheet lined with parchment paper. Cook for 15 minutes or until tender.

3. add mix-ins & serve

Serve simple, or with tasty mix-ins. Puree, mash, or dice according to your baby's stage.

simply pear puree
6 months +

Puree the pear with breast milk, formula, or water in a food processor until smooth and soupy.

pear-apple puree

7 months +

MIX-INS

1 small apple, peeled and chopped

Cook the apple with the pear. Transfer the apple and pear to a food processor and puree until smooth.

pear-avocado puree

8 months +

MIX-INS

½ avocado

Cut the avocado in half and remove the seed. Scoop out the flesh, and then place in a food processor with the pear. Puree until smooth with tiny lumps.

banana-pear infant cereal

9 months +

MIX-INS

1 banana, peeled

¼ cup homemade oat or rice infant cereal

Start by bringing ¾ cups of water to a boil in a small saucepan. Reduce the heat to low and slowly pour in the oat infant cereal. Keep stirring until the cereal is fully mixed into the water. Cook for 5 minutes, or until thickened, stirring occasionally. Meanwhile, place the banana and pears in a food processor and puree to form a soft, lumpy puree. Combine the fruit and oat cereal together in a small bowl.

pear-raisin puree

10 months +

MIX-INS

¼ cup raisins

¼ cup breast milk, formula, or water

Place the raisins in a bowl. Pour enough hot water over the raisins to barely cover them. Let them sit until plump (about 5 minutes). Transfer the raisins and pears to a food processor. Pulse to create a chunky puree.

pear-butternut squash puree

11 months +

MIX-INS

½ cup cubed butternut squash

2 tablespoons breast milk, formula, or water (optional)

Peel the skin off the squash and cut it into cubes (or use frozen butternut squash cubes). Fill ½ cup. Cook fresh butternut squash (microwave for 5–10 minutes, steam for 12 minutes, boil for 13 minutes, or roast at 400°F for 30 minutes). Cook frozen squash according to the package directions. When the pear and squash are cool enough to handle, finely chop into small chunks. Serve 4–5 pieces at a time as finger food, or pulse in a food processor with breast milk, formula, or water to create a chunky puree.

raspberries and pears

12 months +

MIX-INS

½ cup raspberries

Finely dice the raspberries and pears and serve a little in a small bowl as finger food.

---

roasted pears with honey

preparation time: 5 minutes

cook time: 15 minutes

2 pears, halved

cinnamon

2 tablespoons honey

1 tablespoon butter, diced

vanilla ice cream and granola for serving

Preheat the oven to 425°F. Line a baking sheet with aluminum foil and spray with cooking spray.

Cut both pears in half, and then scoop out the seeds and core with a spoon or melon baller. Place the pears on the baking sheet cut side up. Sprinkle with cinnamon, drizzle with honey, and dot with butter.

Bake for 15 minutes, until the pears are fork tender. Serve each pear with a scoop of ice cream and a handful of granola.

walnut pear salad

preparation time: 10 minutes

3 cups mixed greens

½ cup walnuts, chopped

1 pear, sliced

raspberry balsamic dressing

Toss the greens, walnuts, and pears together in a large bowl. Top with just enough dressing to moisten the greens. Divide the salad into two serving bowls.

pears with cream cheese and raisins

preparation time: 5 minutes

2 pears

⅓ cup whipped cream cheese

⅛ cup raisins

Cut the pears in half and remove the core and seeds. Spread the cream cheese on the pear halves, and top with raisins.

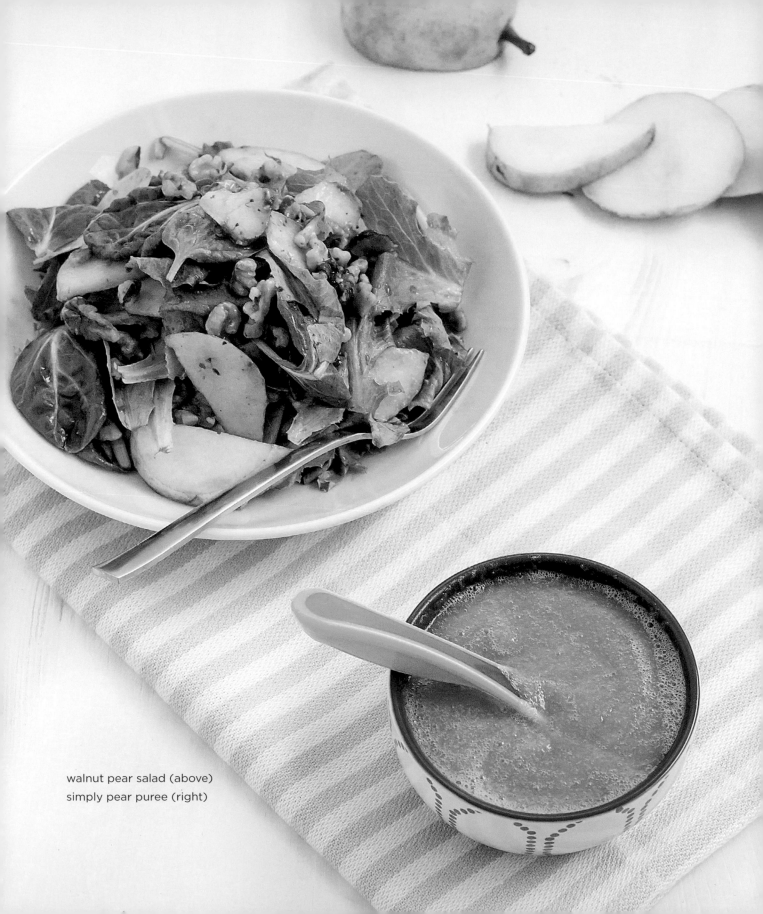

walnut pear salad (above)
simply pear puree (right)

pineapples

Pineapples are high in fiber, copper, and vitamins B and C. These nutrients promote healthy skin and bones, reduce inflammation, and speed the healing of bruises, sprains, and other wounds. They also boost your immune system, promote a healthy heart, and reduce the risk of certain cancers.

pineapple baby food

START WITH ¼ cup pineapple

1. prep

On a cutting board, lay one pineapple on its side. Use a knife to cut off the top and bottom. Stand the pineapple up and carefully trim off the skin from all around the pineapple. Check the pineapple cylinder for any remaining divots and trim those off. Cut into thick slices, carefully removing the core on each slice. Cut the pineapple into chunks.

 Some grocery stores sell fresh-cut pineapple. This is a great option to cut down your preparation time. If you can't find pre-prepared pineapple, you can substitute with frozen pineapple for baby's food, or canned pineapple for you.

Pineapple is very acidic, so you may want to mix it with other food for your baby.

2. add mix-ins and serve

pineapple cottage cheese
11 months +

MIX-INS

½ cup small curd, full-fat cottage cheese

....

Mince pineapple. Place cottage cheese in a small bowl. Then stir in ¼ cup of minced pineapple, reserving the rest for another snack.

baby's first stir-fry
12 months +

MIX-INS

¼ cup cooked chicken, diced

⅛ cup cooked red pepper, diced

2 tablespoons cooked rice

....

This dish is meant to be paired with the adult recipe that follows. Dice the pineapple, chicken, and red pepper. Place in a small bowl and stir in rice.

pineapple cottage cheese

preparation time: 3 minutes

New moms need quick, quality break-fasts to fuel their busy days, and cottage cheese does just that.

¼ cup pineapple, diced

1 cup cottage cheese

whole wheat crackers

Dice pineapple. Spoon the cottage cheese into a serving bowl and top with pineapple. Use the crackers as your utensil to scoop up the cottage cheese and pineapple.

mandarin chicken stir-fry with pineapple

preparation time: 10 minutes

cook time: 10 minutes

½ cup brown or white rice

2 tablespoons canola oil

1 cup pineapple chunks

2 chicken breasts, cut into ½-inch slices

¾ cup red bell pepper, chopped

½ cup frozen sugar snap peas

½ cup store-bought mandarin stir-fry sauce (I use the Panda Express brand)

¼ cup roasted cashews

Follow the package instructions and start cooking the rice. Meanwhile, chop the chicken and peppers and thaw the sugar snap peas.

When the rice has 10 minutes left, heat the oil in a sauté pan over medium-high heat. Add the chicken, peppers, and sugar snap peas. Cook until the chicken juices run clear and the vegetables are nearly tender (about 7 minutes).

Stir in the sauce and pineapple, and cook until the sauce boils. Serve the stir-fry over rice and top with cashews.

pineapple casserole

preparation time: 10 minutes

cook time: 50 minutes

8 slices of white bread

1 (20-ounce) can of crushed pineapple

½ cup butter, melted

¾ cup sugar

4 eggs

1 tablespoon lemon juice

¼ teaspoon nutmeg

Preheat the oven to 350°F. Butter an 8 × 8 baking dish.

Place the bread in a tall stack on a cutting board. Then use a knife to cut off the crust. Discard the crust pieces and cut the bread into cubes.

In a large bowl, whisk together the pineapple, butter, sugar, eggs, lemon juice, and nutmeg until combined. Stir in the bread.

Pour the pineapple and bread mixture into the prepared baking dish. Cook uncovered for 50 minutes.

plantains

Plantains are a staple food in many Caribbean countries. If you've never cooked plantains before, you'll find they are low in sugar yet naturally sweet tasting. They are an excellent source of fiber, potassium, copper, magnesium, phosphorus, as well as vitamins A, B, and C. These nutrients are important for cardiovascular and bone health, metabolism, immunity, and eye function.

 Plantains can be found in three different ripening stages. As plantains ripen, they become sweet, changing color from green to yellow to black. The green ones are the least ripe, and are similar in taste and texture to potatoes. Buy blackened plantains for baby food recipes. They are fully ripe and soft, and easy to digest. If you can't find black plantains, buy green or yellow ones and let them ripen on your counter for one-to-two weeks.

 Unlike bananas, plantains need to be cooked before eating.

plantain baby food

START WITH 2 black plantains

1. cook

There are several ways to cook plantains.

MICROWAVE

cook time: 2 minutes

Slit each side of the plantains, and wrap them in a paper towel. Place the plantains in the microwave and cook for 2 minutes, or until soft. Cut them in half and pop out from the skin.

BOIL

cook time: 10 minutes

Fill half of a large pot with water and bring to a boil. Cut the plantain in half width-wise. Place the plantain halves in the boiling water. Cover and cook for 10 minutes. Remove from the water and pop the plantain out from the skin.

GRILL

cook time: 5 minutes

Heat a grill to 350°F, or a grill pan to medium. Cut in half, and then place face down on the grill. Cook until soft, about 5 minutes. Use a spoon to scoop out the plantain.

 Under-ripe plantains will take longer to cook.

2. add mix-ins & serve

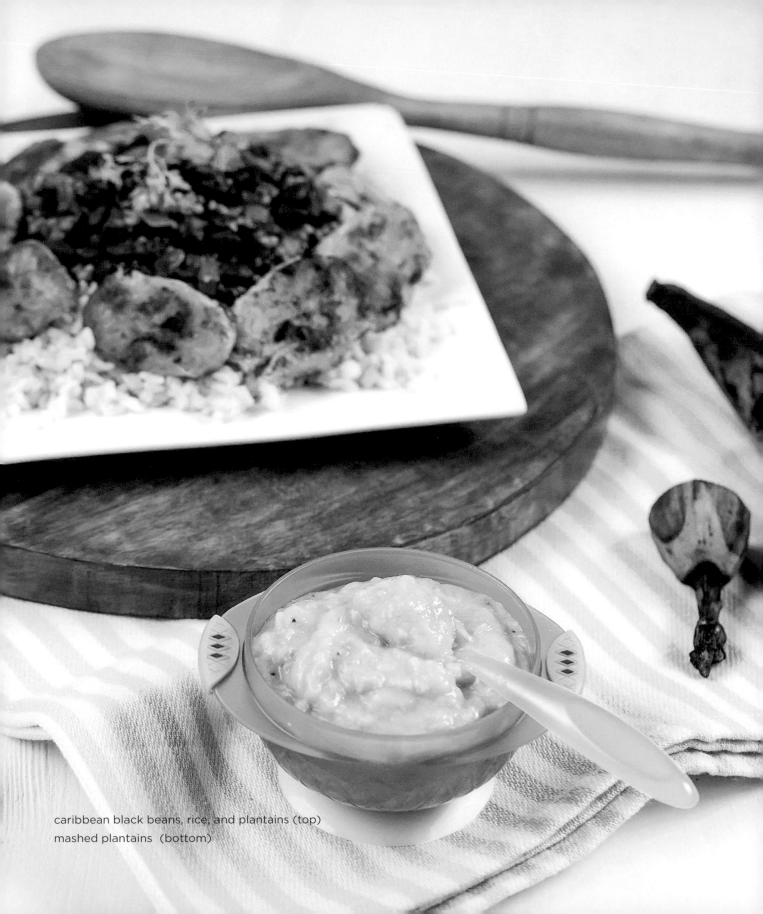

caribbean black beans, rice, and plantains (top)
mashed plantains (bottom)

simply plantain puree

7 months +

MIX-INS

½ cup breast milk, formula, or water

Puree the plantain in a food processor with the breast milk, formula, or water until smooth.

plantain-pumpkin puree

8 months +

MIX-INS

1 cup chopped pumpkin

1 cup breast milk, formula, or water

Steam the pumpkin until tender (5 minutes in the microwave with 1 tablespoon of water, or 12 minutes stovetop). Puree the pumpkin and plantains in a food processor with breast milk, formula, or water until smooth.

mashed plantains

9 months +

MIX-INS

3 tablespoons breast milk, formula, or water

In a medium bowl, mash the plantains and breast milk, formula, or water with a fork (or pulse in a food processor) until thick and creamy with some small lumps.

plantain-peach puree

10 months +

MIX-INS

1 large peach

⅓ cup breast milk, formula, or water

Slice a peach in half to remove the pit. Cook the peach until tender (microwave for 2 minutes, steam for 5 minutes, or boil for 8–10 minutes). When the peach is cool to the touch, peel off the skin. Next, place the plantain, peach, and breast milk, formula, or water in the bowl of a food processor and puree to a chunky consistency.

plantain-avocado puree

11 months +

MIX-INS

1 large avocado

½ cup breast milk, formula, or water

Halve the avocado and remove the pit. Scoop the avocado flesh into a medium bowl. Mash the plantains, avocado, and breast milk, formula, or water until combined (or place in a food processor) to create a chunky puree.

beans, rice, and plantains

12 months +

MIX-INS

¼ cup cooked brown rice

¼ cup prepared black beans

This recipe is meant to be paired with the adult recipe that follows. Stir the cooked rice and black beans together in a small bowl. Lightly smash the beans with a fork. Dice the plantains into bite-sized pieces, measuring out ¼ cup. Store the remaining plantains in the refrigerator for another meal. Add the plantains to the bowl and stir.

mama recipes

plantain avocado salad

preparation time: 5 minutes

2 ripe plantains

1 avocado

Slit the side of each plantain and wrap them in paper towels. Place the plantains in the microwave and cook for 2 minutes, or until soft. Cut them in half and pop out from the skin.

Dice the avocado and plantains and stir together. Eat immediately or serve chilled.

roasted sea salt plantains

preparation time: 5 minutes

cook time: 30 minutes

2 plantains

coarse sea salt

Preheat oven to 350°F. Cover a baking sheet with aluminum foil and lightly spray with olive oil cooking spray.

Peel the plantains, and then cut into ½-inch slices.

Arrange the plantain slices in a single layer on the prepared baking sheet and sprinkle with sea salt. Spray a quick mist of cooking spray over the plantains cook for 15 minutes. Flip and cook for another 15 minutes, or until slightly crispy and golden brown on both sides.

caribbean black beans, rice, and plantains

preparation time: 10 minutes

cook time: 40 minutes

1 cup white or brown rice

1 (15-ounce) can of black beans or 1½ cups of prepared black beans

⅓ cup white onion, diced

½ teaspoon chili powder

2 garlic cloves, minced

1 tablespoon olive oil (optional)

2 tablespoons canola oil

2 black plantains, peeled and sliced into ½-inch pieces

Follow the instructions on the package to start cooking the rice.

In a small saucepan, add the beans, diced onions, chili powder, and minced garlic. If using fresh beans, add 1 tablespoon of olive oil to the saucepan. Cook on medium-high until the beans are hot and the onions begin to wilt. Then decrease the heat to low until you are ready to serve.

Start cooking the plantains when the rice has about 10 minutes left. Heat the canola oil in a sauté pan over medium heat. Wet your hands and flick a few drops of water onto the pan. When the water sizzles in the oil, add as many plantain slices as can fit comfortably in the pan. Depending on the size of your pan, you may need to cook in two batches. Cook the plantains until golden brown (about 1–2 minutes per side). Line a plate with paper towels and place the plantains on top to absorb excess grease.

Lightly mash the beans in the saucepan and serve over rice with plantains on the side.

caramelized plantains

total time: 10 minutes

2 ripe plantains

2 tablespoons brown sugar

1 tablespoon butter

Cut the plantains in half lengthwise, and then remove the plantain from the peel and cut into ½-inch slices.

Heat a nonstick skillet over medium-high heat, and add the butter. When melted, add the plantains and brown sugar.

Sauté until the plantains caramelize, about 3–4 minutes.

plums and prunes

Plums are a good source of antioxidants, fiber, potassium, copper, and vitamins B, C, and K. Are you or baby having digestion problems? Try eating some plums or prunes. They are known to help relieve constipation, promote healthy bowel movements, and generally improve digestion.

Plums also help fight harmful free radicals in the body. This can reduce the risk for breast cancer and diabetes.

Plums are in season during the summer, but they may not be available in grocery stores the rest of the year. If they aren't available, try the dried version, prunes. Like dried figs, prunes contain more nutrients than their fresh counterpart, and even more antioxidants than blueberries. Choose prunes that are made without added sugar or preservatives.

plum and prune baby food

START WITH 4 fresh plums or 1 cup pitted prunes

1. prep

Wash fresh plums, and then halve and remove the pit. Sometimes you can use your hands to remove the peel of very ripe plums. Otherwise, keep the peel on. After you make a puree, push it through a fine mesh strainer to separate from the skin.

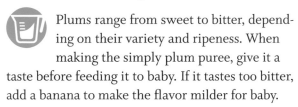

Plums range from sweet to bitter, depending on their variety and ripeness. When making the simply plum puree, give it a taste before feeding it to baby. If it tastes too bitter, add a banana to make the flavor milder for baby.

2. cook

Plums don't need to be cooked. Choose your cooking method for prunes.

MICROWAVE

cook time: 3 minutes

Place the prunes in a microwave-safe bowl. Cover with water and microwave until plump.

STEEP

cook time: 5 minutes

Place the prunes in a bowl. Pour enough hot water over the prunes to barely cover them. Let them sit until plump. Save the excess (nutrition packed) cooking water to help thin out baby's purees.

3. add mix-ins & serve

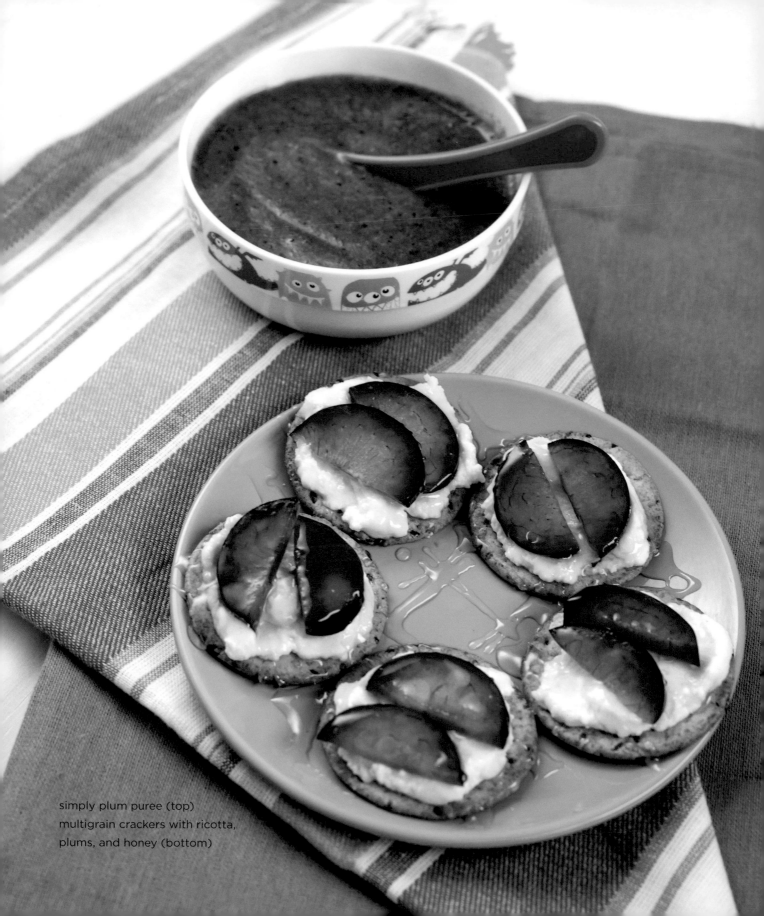

simply plum puree (top)
multigrain crackers with ricotta,
plums, and honey (bottom)

simply plum puree

7 months +

MIX-INS

4 tablespoons breast milk, formula, or cooking water (for prunes only)

Place plums (or prunes) in a food processor. If using prunes, add breast milk, formula, or cooking water. Puree until smooth.

pear-prune puree

8 months +

MIX-INS

1 ripe pear, peeled, cored, and quartered

½ cup prune cooking water or breast milk, formula, or water (reduce to 1 tablespoon for plums)

Cook the pear until tender (microwave for 2 minutes, steam for 4 minutes, boil for 10 minutes, or bake for 20 minutes at 425°F). Puree the prunes or plums, pear, and breast milk, formula, or water in a food processor until smooth and thick.

plum, peach, and banana puree

9 months +

MIX-INS

1 peach, halved and pitted

2 bananas, peeled

1 tablespoon breast milk, formula, or water (add an additional ⅓ cup for prunes)

Cook the peach until tender (microwave for 2 minutes, steamed on the stove for 5 minutes, or roast for 20 minutes at 425°F). When cool enough to the touch, slice or peel off the skin. Place the plums or prunes, peach, banana, and breast milk, formula, or water in a food processor and whirl to form a soft, lumpy puree.

carrots and prunes

10 months +

MIX-INS

1¾ cups baby carrots, or peeled and chopped carrots

¼ cup breast milk, formula, or cooking water

Cook the carrots until tender (microwave for 3–6 minutes, steam or boil for 7–9 minutes, or roast for 25 minutes at 400°F). Transfer carrots, prunes, and breast milk, formula, or water into the bowl of a food processor. Pulse to finely dice and combine.

prune yogurt

11 months +

MIX-INS

½ cup plain, full-fat yogurt

1 tablespoon ground flax seed

Let the prunes cool, and then place ¼ cup prunes, yogurt, and ground flax seed in a food processor. Puree until smooth.

apple, prunes, and chicken

12 months +

MIX-INS

¼ cup boneless, skinless chicken breast

¼ apple, peeled and halved

Cook the chicken through (sauté for 10 minutes, poach for 10 minutes, grill for 12 minutes, or bake for 15 minutes at 375°F). Meanwhile, cut the apple in half and remove the core. Cook the apple until tender (microwave for 3–4 minutes, steam for 12 minutes, or bake for 15 minutes at 375°F). Cut the chicken, apples, and prunes into pea-sized cubes. Serve as finger food or whirl into a chunky puree.

mama recipes

apple, prune, and sunflower seed salad

preparation time: 10 minutes

4 cups mixed greens

1 apple, sliced

2 tablespoons sunflower seeds

½ cup walnuts, chopped

⅓ cup pitted prunes, diced

apple or raspberry vinaigrette

In a large bowl, add the greens, then the apple slices, sunflower seeds, walnuts, and prunes. Season with salt and pepper and drizzle with vinaigrette.

multigrain crackers with ricotta, plums, and honey

preparation time: 10 minutes

This grown-up snack satisfies sweet cravings, while offering fiber and protein to help boost your energy.

multigrain crackers

¼ cup ricotta cheese

1 plum, sliced

honey

Spread crackers with ricotta and a few plum or prune slices. Drizzle with honey.

chicken with apple-prune stuffing

preparation time: 10 minutes

cook time: 30 minutes

2 large chicken breasts

1 cup seasoned stuffing mix

¼ cup prunes, finely diced

½ apple, peeled and diced

¼ cup chopped pecans

Preheat the oven to 350°F. Spray a baking dish with cooking spray.

Cook the stuffing mix as directed on the box, and then stir in the chopped apples, prunes, and pecans.

Place the chicken breasts on a cutting board and cover with plastic wrap. Using a mallet, pound the chicken to ¼-inch. Place a mound of stuffing on each breast and roll it up. Place the chicken seam side down on the baking dish.

Cover with aluminum foil and bake for 20–30 minutes or until cooked through.

vegetables

asparagus

Asparagus is an aphrodisiac so it boosts your sex drive (nothing like vegetables to get you in the mood). After giving birth, many women, especially those who are nursing, have lower libidos than before they were pregnant. So if you're looking to heighten your desire, try eating more asparagus!

Asparagus is also an excellent source of vitamin K and folate. It promotes healthy bones and may prevent heart disease and certain cancers.

asparagus baby food

START WITH 1 pound of asparagus

1. prep

Wash the asparagus, then cut off the tough, woody stem, and chop into 2-inch long pieces.

2. cook

There are a variety of ways to cook asparagus.

MICROWAVE

cook time: 2 minutes

Place the asparagus in a microwave-safe baking dish with 1 tablespoon of water. Microwave until very tender, about 2–4 minutes.

BOIL

cook time: 3 minutes

Fill half of a medium saucepan with water and bring to a boil over medium-high heat. Add the asparagus, and cook until very tender, about 3–5 minutes. Drain the asparagus in a colander.

STEAM

cook time: 4 minutes

Set up a steamer basket in a medium pot and add enough water to reach just below the basket. Bring the water to a boil. Cover and steam the asparagus until very tender, 4–5 minutes.

ROAST

cook time: 15 minutes

Preheat the oven to 400°F. Spread the asparagus in a single layer on a baking sheet. Toss in olive oil and roast for 15 minutes.

3. add mix-ins & serve

Serve simply, or with tasty mix-ins. Puree or dice according to your baby's stage.

simply asparagus puree

9 months +

MIX-INS

2 tablespoons breast milk, formula, or water

Transfer the asparagus and breast milk, formula, or water to a food processor and blitz to create a soft puree with small bits.

apple-asparagus puree

10 months +

MIX-INS

2 apples, peeled and chopped

1 tablespoon breast milk, formula, or water

Cook apples until tender (microwave for 3 minutes, steam for 12 minutes or bake for 15 minutes at 375°F). Place the cooked asparagus, apple, and breast milk, formula, or water in the bowl of a food processor and pulse until finely diced.

asparagus and carrot medley

11 months +

MIX-INS

1 cup baby carrots, or peeled and chopped carrots

2 tablespoons breast milk, formula, or water

Cook the carrots until tender (microwave for 3 minutes, steam or boil for 7 minutes, sauté in butter for 10 minutes, or roast for 25 minutes at 400°F). Transfer the asparagus, carrots, and breast milk, formula, or water to a food processor and blitz until finely diced.

asparagus with linguine

12 months +

MIX-INS

3 linguine noodles, cooked

This recipe is meant to be paired with the adult recipe that follows. Cut the linguine into ¼ inch pieces. Slice the asparagus into pea-sized pieces. In a small bowl, stir a few tablespoons of pasta and asparagus (reserving the rest for another meal). Serve as finger food.

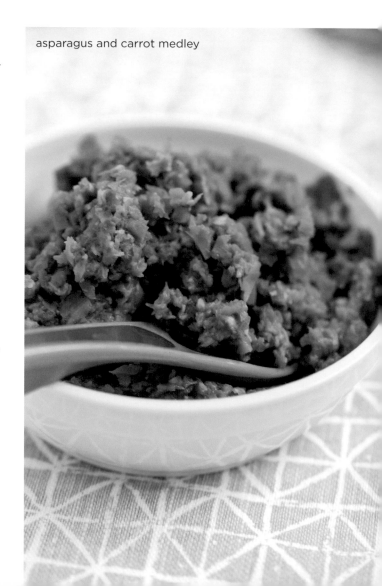

asparagus and carrot medley

grilled asparagus with bacon

preparation time: 5 minutes

cook time: 10 minutes

10 large asparagus, trimmed (a little under ½ pound)

3 bacon strips

2 skewers

Preheat the grill to 350°F.

Place the asparagus in a row on a cutting board. To make a rack of asparagus, insert a skewer near the top of the asparagus, piercing through all 10 pieces. Use another skewer to thread all of the asparagus near the bottom.

Wrap the rack of asparagus with the bacon, placing them side by side across the asparagus, then tuck in the ends.

Place the skewers on the grill and cook for about 5 minutes, then flip. Continue to cook until the asparagus is tender and the bacon is crispy and cooked.

Use tongs or a kitchen glove to slide the asparagus off the skewers and onto the serving plates.

roasted asparagus with pine nuts

preparation time: 5 minutes

cook time: 10 minutes

½ pound asparagus

2 tablespoons olive oil

¼ cup pine nuts

2 garlic cloves, minced

Preheat the oven to 450°F.

Place the asparagus on a baking sheet in a single layer. Drizzle with olive oil, and then top with pine nuts and garlic. Season with salt and pepper.

Roast for 5 minutes, then flip. Cook another 5 minutes or until crisp.

shrimp linguine with lemon-parsley sauce

preparation time: 15 minutes

cook time: 15 minutes

½ **box of linguine**

3 **tablespoons olive oil**

3 **garlic cloves, minced**

½ **cup onion, diced**

20–25 **medium shrimp, peeled and deveined**

1½ **cups asparagus cut into 1½-inch pieces**

for the sauce:

¼ **cup reserved pasta water**

1 **tablespoon butter**

½ **tablespoon dried parsley**

2 **tablespoons fresh lemon juice**

Bring a pot of water to a boil and add pasta. Cook for about 10 minutes, or until al dente. Scoop out ¼ cup of the pasta water and drain the rest.

Meanwhile, heat the olive oil in a skillet and add the garlic, onions, shrimp, and asparagus. Cover and cook for 3–5 minutes, or until the shrimp is cooked and the asparagus is tender. Stir in the reserved pasta water, butter, parsley, and lemon juice. Serve over linguine.

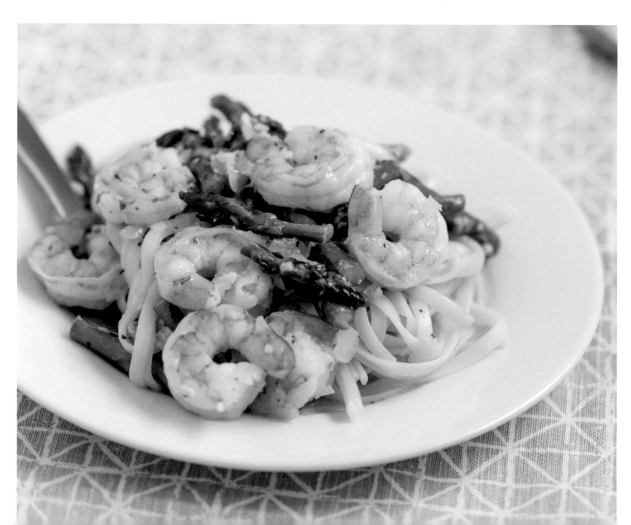

avocados

Though technically a fruit, avocados are often used like a vegetable. They are an excellent source of potassium and fiber, as well as vitamins C, E, and K. These nutrients strengthen the immune system, soften the skin, and keep your eyes and heart healthy.

As if this wasn't enough, avocado also contains healthy monounsaturated fats, which may help lower bad LDL cholesterol (the type of cholesterol that contributes to plaque build up) and reduce risk of stroke and heart disease. They even contain some protein!

avocado baby food

START WITH 1 avocado

1. prep

Use a small paring knife to cut the avocado in half. First cut lengthwise down one side, and then move the knife carefully around the entire fruit, avoiding the large seed in the center. Gently twist the halves apart in opposite directions. Use a large spoon to remove the seed, and then scoop the avocado out of the skin.

2. add mix-ins & serve

simply avocado puree

6 months +

MIX-INS

½ cup breast milk, formula, or water

Puree the avocado and breast milk, formula, or water in a food processor until smooth and soupy.

avocado-banana puree

7 months +

MIX-INS

1 banana

¼ cup breast milk, formula, or water

Peel the banana and place it in a food processor with the avocado and breast milk, formula, or water. Puree until smooth and soupy.

avocado and infant rice cereal

8 months +

MIX-INS

¼ cup homemade brown rice cereal

2 tablespoons breast milk, formula, or water

Bring 1 cup of water to a boil. While whisking constantly, sprinkle in ¼ cup of ground brown rice. Continue to whisk for 1 minute. Reduce heat to a simmer and stir occasionally for 15 minutes, or until thickened. Meanwhile, puree ½ the avocado until smooth, then stir into the cooked rice cereal with the breast milk, formula, or water.

avocado-egg yolk puree

9 months +

MIX-INS

4 egg yolks from hard boiled eggs

2 tablespoon breast milk, formula, or water

Measure ½ avocado (reserving the rest for another meal). Using a fork, mash the avocado and egg yolk together, or puree in a food processor to form a thick puree with tiny lumps.

cool avocado and cucumber

10 months +

MIX-INS

¾ cucumber, peeled and chopped

Peel the cucumber and cut in half lengthwise. Use a spoon to remove the seeds in the center, and then cut into chunks. Place the cucumber and avocado in a food processor and pulse to finely dice and combine.

avocado and chicken

11 months +

MIX-INS

½ cup chopped boneless chicken breast

Cook chicken until no longer pink (poach for 10 minutes, grill for 12 minutes, sauté for 10 minutes, or bake for 10–15 minutes at 375°F). Finely dice the chicken and ½ cup avocado, and then serve a few pieces at a time as finger food. Save the leftovers in the refrigerator for another meal.

avocado toast

12 months +

MIX-INS

1 slice whole wheat bread

Place ½ of the avocado in a bowl. Use a fork to mash together until smooth. Meanwhile, toast the bread. Spread some of the avocado on the toast. Then cut off the crust and cut into slices a little hand can hold.

If your baby doesn't care for the taste of avocado on its own, make avocado cream cheese toast instead. Mash equal parts avocado and whipped full-fat cream cheese, then spread it on toast!

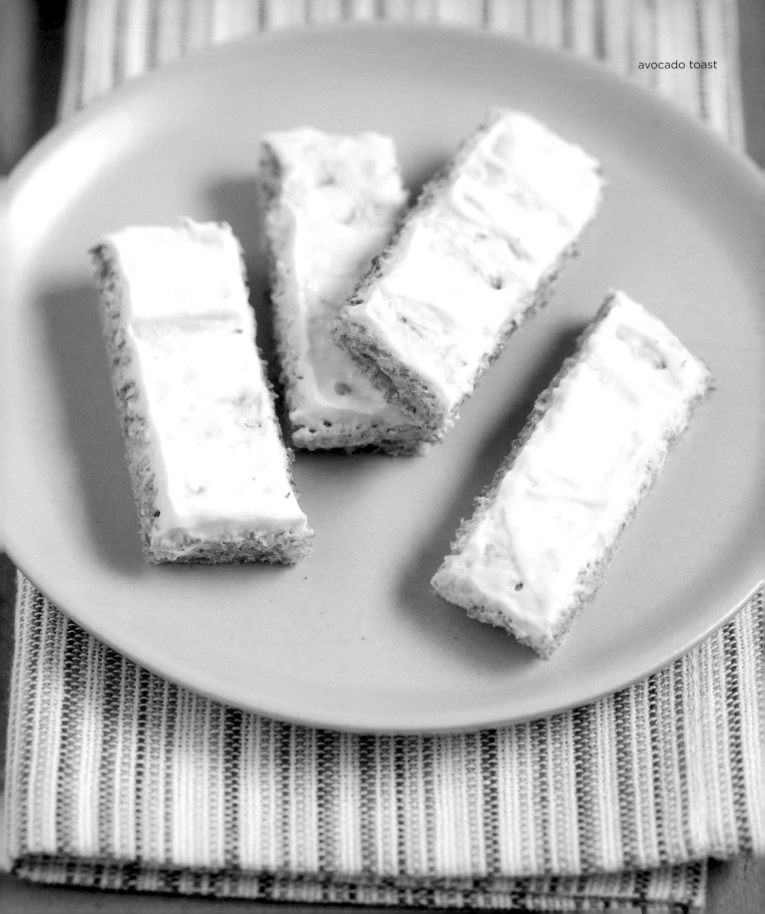

avocado toast

spicy avocado toast

total time: 5 minutes

4 slices whole-grain bread

1 avocado

Sriracha hot sauce

Toast the bread. Meanwhile, mash the avocado in a small bowl. Spread the toast with avocado and drizzle with Sriracha.

cobb salad

total time: 10 minutes

To save prep time, get the tomatoes, avocado and egg from the grocery store salad bar, then add them to the top of your salad right before serving.

4 cups fresh spinach or lettuce

½ cup cherry tomatoes, halved

½ avocado, peeled and chopped

¼ cup shredded cheddar cheese

2 hard-boiled eggs, cut into wedges

½ cup Italian croutons

ranch or blue cheese dressing

Italian bread

In a large bowl, toss the greens, tomatoes, avocado, and cheese together. Divide between two serving bowls.

Top each salad with eggs, croutons, and dressing. Serve a few slices of bread on the side.

avocado and lime shrimp tacos

total time: 25 minutes

4 tomatillos

1 tablespoon canola oil

15 shrimp, shelled and deveined

¾ cup of frozen sliced bell peppers

¼ teaspoon lime juice

4 flour tortillas

1 avocado, peeled and sliced

Fill a medium pot with water and bring to a boil. Add the tomatillos. Cook for about 5 minutes. Then use a slotted spoon to remove from the pot. When cool to the touch, peel off the husks, and dice.

Meanwhile, heat the canola oil over medium heat on a nonstick skillet. Add the shrimp and peppers. Cook until the shrimp are pink and cooked through and the peppers are tender and crisp (about 5 minutes).

Season shrimp with salt and pepper and a few drops of lime juice.

Heat tortillas in a microwave until warm (about 10 seconds). Assemble tortillas by adding shrimp, peppers, avocado, and tomatillos.

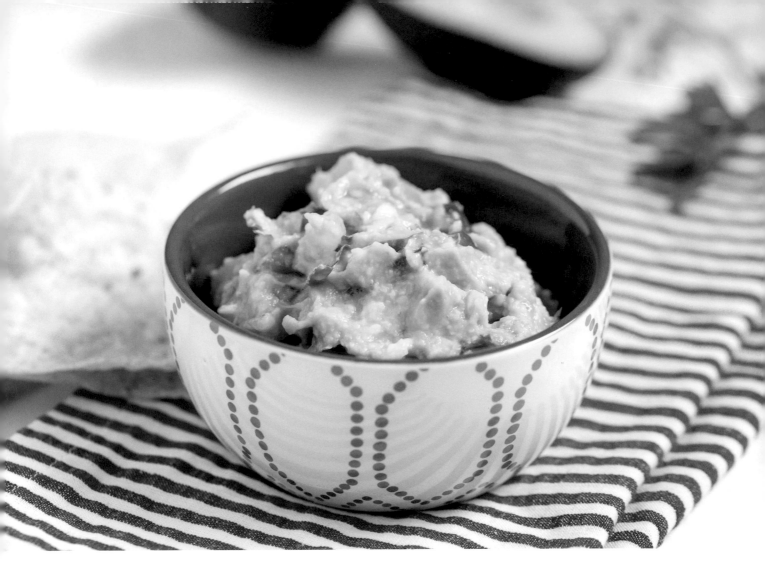

guacamole

total time: 15 minutes

1 hass avocado, halved, pitted, and peeled

½ plum tomato, finely chopped

⅓ cup white onion, finely chopped

1 tablespoon each fresh parsley and cilantro, chopped

1 tablespoon lime juice

Scoop the avocado into a medium bowl. Stir in the tomato, onion, herbs, and lime juice. Season with salt and pepper.

Serve as a dip with tortilla chips or veggie sticks, or as a condiment to tacos, fajitas, or quesadillas.

avocados

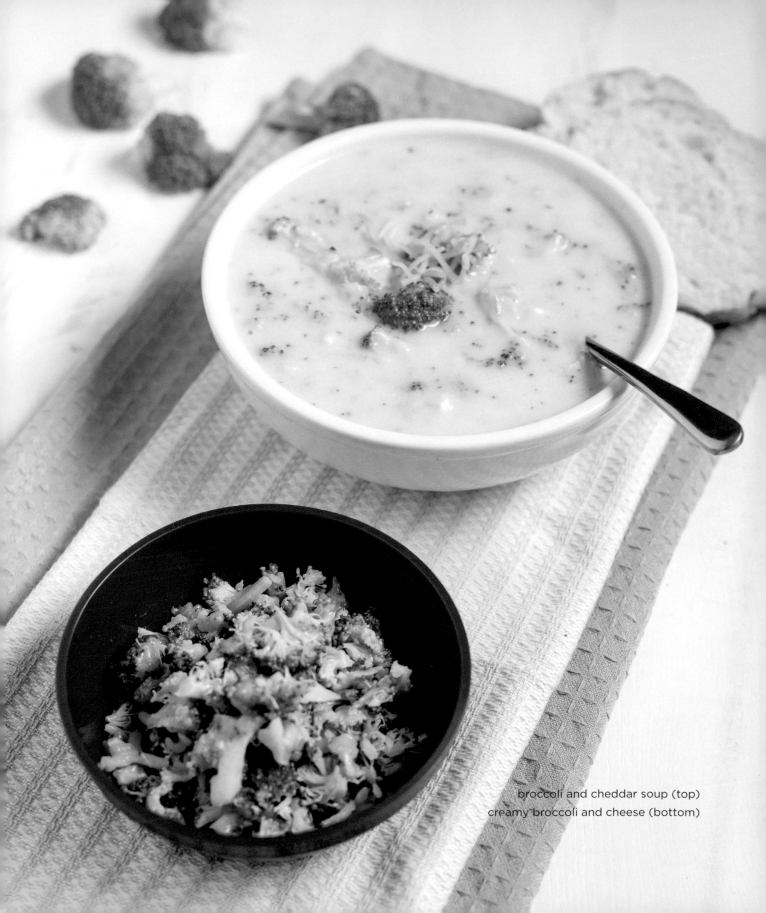

broccoli and cheddar soup (top)
creamy broccoli and cheese (bottom)

broccoli

Broccoli is rich in vitamins C and K, folic acid, calcium, and fiber. It helps detoxify the body and prevent cancerous cells from forming. Broccoli promotes healthy growth and development in children and strong bones and teeth. It also decreases symptoms of PMS and boosts mood.

broccoli baby food

START WITH 1 heaping cup of fresh or frozen broccoli florets and stems

1. prep

If using fresh broccoli, cut off the end stalk of 1 head. Chop into florets, cutting out and discarding any brown, wilted, mushy, or deteriorated stems or sprouts. Wash thoroughly.

2. cook

Cook frozen broccoli as directed on the bag. If using fresh broccoli, choose from the following cooking options.

MICROWAVE

cook time: 2 minutes

Place the broccoli in a microwave-safe bowl with 1 tablespoon of water. Cover and microwave for 2–5 minutes or until very tender.

BOIL

cook time: 5 minutes

Fill half of a medium saucepan with water and bring to a boil over medium-high heat. Add the broccoli, and cook until very tender, about 5 minutes. Drain the broccoli in a colander.

STEAM

cook time: 6 minutes

Set up a steamer basket in a medium pot. Add enough water so it reaches just below the basket.

Bring to a boil. Cover and steam the broccoli for about 6 minutes, or until tender.

ROAST

cook time: 10 minutes

Cover a baking sheet with aluminum foil. Lightly spray with olive oil cooking spray. Spread the broccoli florets and stems on the baking sheet in a single layer. Roast at 425°F for 10 minutes, or until tender.

3. add mix-ins & serve

Serve on its own or with tasty mix-ins. Puree or dice according to your baby's stage.

simply broccoli puree

9 months +

MIX-INS

2 tablespoons breast milk, formula, or water

Puree the cooked broccoli and breast milk, formula, or water in a food processor to make a thick puree with tiny lumps.

creamy broccoli and cheese

10 months +

MIX-INS

¼ cup shredded cheddar cheese

2 tablespoons breast milk, formula, or water

Place the broccoli, cheese, and breast milk, formula, or water in a food processor, and puree to form a finely chopped mixture.

chicken and broccoli

11 months +

MIX-INS

⅓ cup diced chicken

Cook chicken until no longer pink (sauté for 10 minutes, poach for 15 minutes, grill for 12 minutes, or bake for 15 minutes at 375°F). Cut the chicken into pea-sized cubes, and the broccoli into small pieces. In a small bowl, stir the broccoli and chicken together. Serve as finger food.

broccoli and egg yolk

12 months +

MIX-INS

3 hard-boiled eggs

Remove the shells and rinse the eggs in water to remove any small bits of shell. Peel the egg white open, take out the yolk, and place it on a cutting board. Cut the egg yolk and ¼ cup of broccoli into small chunks. Serve as finger food.

chicken-broccoli ranch rice bowl

preparation time: 5 minutes

cook time: 20 minutes

This recipe is a family favorite. It's quick and easy to prepare, and we almost always have the ingredients on hand. Plus, the balance of healthy chicken and broccoli and indulgent cheese and ranch make it a meal we almost always crave.

1 cup white rice

1 tablespoon canola oil

2 chicken breasts, chopped

1 tablespoon Worcestershire sauce

2 cups broccoli, chopped

½ cup shredded cheddar cheese

ranch dressing

Begin cooking the rice as directed on the bag.

When the rice has about 15 minutes left, heat the oil in a nonstick skillet over medium-high heat. Add the chicken and cook until browned on one side, then flip. Pour the Worcestershire sauce into the pan, and coat the chicken with the sauce. Finish cooking the chicken through.

Meanwhile, steam the broccoli until tender (2–5 minutes in the microwave or 6 minutes on the stove).

Once the chicken, broccoli, and rice are cooked, start to build your rice bowl! Layer two serving bowls with rice mixed with cheese, chicken, and broccoli. Then top with more cheese. Drizzle with ranch dressing.

beef and broccoli

preparation time: 5 minutes

cook time: 20 minutes

1 tablespoon vegetable oil

¾ pound boneless round steak or top sirloin, sliced

2 cups frozen broccoli florets and stems, thawed

½ cup good-quality teriyaki sauce

⅓ cup salted peanuts

rice for serving

Heat a wok or nonstick skillet over high heat. Add the vegetable oil and beef. Cook for 3 minutes, and then add the broccoli. Cook until the broccoli is tender-crisp and stir in the sauce.

Stir until the mixture thickens and coats the beef and broccoli, about 3 minutes. Serve the stir-fry with rice. Top with salted peanuts for some crunch.

broccoli stromboli

preparation time: 15 minutes

cook time: 20 minutes

This stromboli makes really delicious leftovers (if you can resist not eating the whole thing at once). Reheat in the oven for best results. For meat lovers, add ham, sausage, or pepperoni to the filling.

½ **pound pizza dough**

¾ **cup marinara sauce**

1 **cup broccoli florets, cooked and chopped**

2 **cups shredded mozzarella cheese**

1 **teaspoon Italian seasoning**

1 **egg**

Preheat oven to 450°F and line a baking sheet with parchment paper.

Clean an area of your counter and lightly flour it. Place your pizza dough on the flour and use a rolling pin (or wine bottle) to roll it out into a long, rectangular shape.

Spoon the sauce over the dough, leaving a 1-inch border around the edge. Evenly layer the broccoli on top of the sauce, and then add the cheese. Sprinkle with salt, pepper, and Italian seasoning.

Roll the dough as tight as you can so it forms the shape of a log, then carefully transfer the stromboli to the baking sheet.

Next, make an egg wash to give the stromboli a nice glossy finish. Whisk the egg in a small bowl with 1 tablespoon of water. Then brush it over the top of the stromboli. Sprinkle with salt.

Bake for 20 minutes, or until golden brown.

broccoli and cheddar soup

preparation time: 10 minutes

cook time: 20 minutes

This warm and comforting soup is perfect for cold-weather weekends.

4 **tablespoons butter**

⅓ **cup onion, diced**

⅓ **cup all-purpose flour**

2 **cups chicken stock**

1¾ **cups milk**

4 **cups frozen broccoli florets**

2½ **cups shredded cheese**

In a large pot, melt the butter over medium heat. Add the onion and cook until tender. Stir in the flour, coating the onion. Cook for about 30 seconds, and then add the chicken stock and milk at the same time and stir. Cook over medium heat until the soup is thick. Keep an eye on the pot, making sure it doesn't boil.

Meanwhile, place the broccoli and ¼ cup of water in a microwave-safe bowl. Cover with a paper towel and microwave until tender-crisp. Pour the broccoli into a colander positioned over the sink to drain the water.

Move the pot off the burner, and then stir in the cheese and broccoli. Season with salt and pepper. Taste and add more seasoning if needed. Return the pot to the burner, and let cook on medium-low for 5 minutes to melt the cheese.

brussels sprouts

Brussels sprouts are high in vitamins C and K, folate, manganese, and fiber. This vegetable helps detoxify the body, reduce inflammation, and may help prevent certain cancers, including breast and ovarian. It can also help improve mood and keep skin and hair healthy.

brussels sprout baby food

START WITH 2 cups of fresh or frozen brussels sprouts

1. prep

Wash the brussels sprouts with cold water. Slice off the stems, then remove any of the outer leaves that are blemished, wilted, or yellow.

2. cook

If using frozen brussels sprouts, cook as directed on the package. If using fresh brussels sprouts, choose from the following cooking options.

MICROWAVE

cook time: 2 minutes

Place brussels sprouts in a microwave-safe dish with 1 tablespoon of water. Cover and microwave on high for 2–4 minutes, or until tender.

BOIL

cook time: 5 minutes

Bring a medium pot of water to a boil. Add the brussels sprouts and cook for 5–10 minutes, or until tender.

STEAM

cook time: 8 minutes

Set up a steamer basket in a medium pot and add enough water to reach just below the basket.

Bring to a boil. Cover and steam the brussels sprouts for 8–10 minutes, or until tender.

GRILL

cook time: 10 minutes

Heat a grill to 350°F. Place the brussels sprouts in an aluminum foil pouch sprayed with olive oil, in a metal grill basket, or on skewers. Place on the grill, and cook for 10 minutes, flipping halfway through.

SAUTÉ

cook time: 10 minutes

Cut the brussels sprouts in half. Add a tablespoon of oil to a hot skillet. Then cook for 10 minutes or until tender.

ROAST

cook time: 20 minutes

Preheat oven to 400°F. Line a baking sheet with aluminum foil and spread the brussels sprouts out in a single layer. Roast for 20 minutes, flipping the sprouts halfway through.

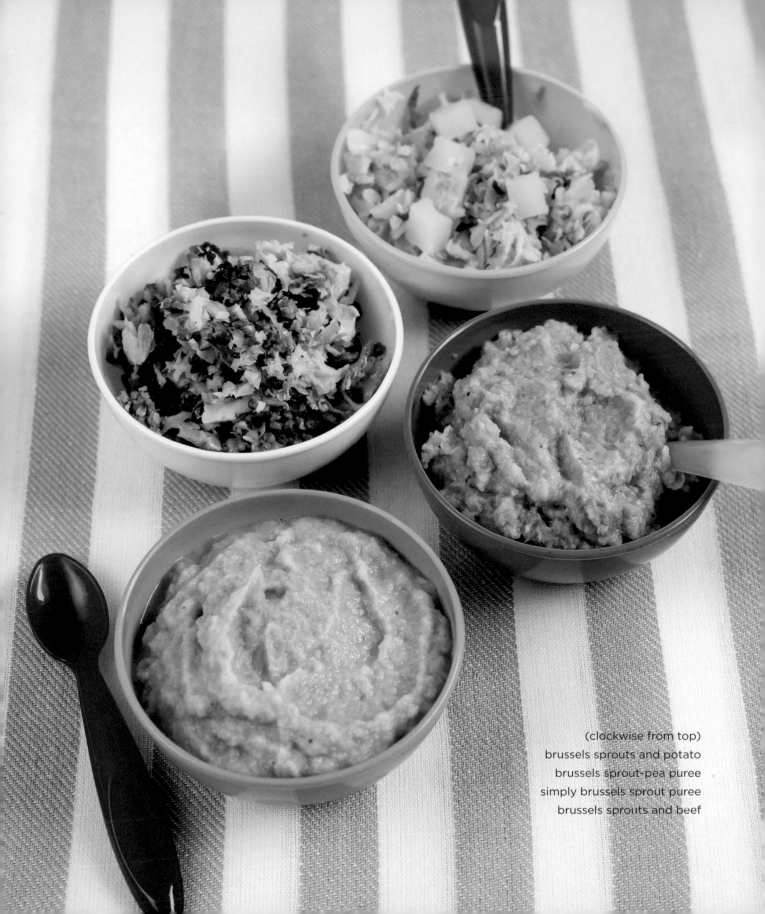

(clockwise from top)
brussels sprouts and potato
brussels sprout-pea puree
simply brussels sprout puree
brussels sprouts and beef

3. add mix-ins & serve

Serve on its own, or with tasty mix-ins. Puree or finely dice according to your baby's stage.

simply brussels sprout puree

8 months +

MIX-INS

½ cup breast milk, formula, or water

Transfer the cooked brussels sprouts and the breast milk, formula, or water to a food processor. Whirl to form a smooth, thick puree.

brussels sprout-pea puree

9 months +

MIX-INS

½ cup peas

½ cup + 2 tablespoons breast milk, formula, or water

Cook the peas until tender, 2 minutes in the microwave, or 3 minutes steamed or boiled. Transfer the peas, cooked brussels sprouts, and breast milk, formula, or water to a food processor. Whirl into a coarse and chunky puree.

brussels sprouts and beef

10 months +

MIX-INS

¼ pound ground beef (1 cup cooked)

Sauté the beef on medium-high in a skillet. Use a spatula to chop up the meat. Cook through. Drain any grease from the pan, and then place in a food processor with the cooked brussels sprouts. Puree until coarse and chunky.

brussels sprouts and potato

11 months +

MIX-INS

1 small potato

Wash the potato, and then use a fork to poke holes all over. Place on a microwave-safe dish and microwave for 9 minutes, or until tender. Cut the potato in half. Then scoop out the insides, discarding the peel. Dice the potato and brussels sprouts into bite-sized pieces. Scatter a few pieces onto baby's tray, adding more as baby eats them.

brussels sprouts with bacon

12 months +

MIX-INS

2 bacon strips

Cook the bacon (microwave for 2 minutes, then increase by 30 seconds until cooked, or cook on the stovetop) until crispy. Dice the bacon and ½ cup cooked brussels sprouts. Serve together in a bowl as finger food.

brussels sprouts with bacon

preparation time: 5 minutes

cook time: 10 minutes

4 bacon strips, chopped

1 tablespoon olive oil

2 cups brussels sprouts, halved

Heat the oil in a sauté pan over medium-high heat. Add the brussels sprouts and bacon, and cook until the bacon is crispy.

Add ¼ cup water to the pan, then cover and cook until the water mostly evaporates and the brussels sprouts are tender, about 5 minutes. Season with salt and pepper.

oven-roasted brussels sprouts

preparation time: 5 minutes

cook time: 40 minutes

2 cups brussels sprouts, halved

1 tablespoon olive oil

sea salt

Preheat the oven to 400°F.

Place the brussels sprouts in a bowl, and toss in olive oil. Cover a rimmed baking sheet with aluminum foil, and then spread the brussels sprouts on the pan in a single layer. Season with coarse sea salt and pepper.

Roast for 20 minutes, then flip and cook for another 20 minutes, or until golden brown on the outside and tender on the inside.

lemon couscous with brussels sprouts

preparation time: 10 minutes

cook time: 15 minutes

1 (5.9 ounce) box of couscous

2 tablespoons olive oil

2 garlic cloves, minced

1½ cups brussels sprouts, trimmed

2 tablespoons lemon juice

Cook the couscous as directed on the box. Meanwhile, mince the garlic and clean and trim the brussels sprouts.

Heat 2 tablespoons of olive oil in a skillet over medium heat. Add the garlic and brussels sprouts and season with salt and pepper. Sauté until cara-melized and tender (about 8–10 minutes), turning the sprouts to sear both sides.

Use a fork to fluff the couscous. Then add the brussels sprouts and lemon juice, stirring to combine.

carrots

Carrots are an excellent source of beta-carotene, which can aid eyesight, promote healthy skin, and help the body fight off colds and infection. Studies have shown that the nutrients in carrots may reduce risk of developing heart disease and breast cancer. Just one small carrot gives you all your recommended daily intake of vitamin A.

 Instead of buying whole carrots, look for baby carrots. They will save you time prepping because they are already peeled, chopped, and ready to go!

carrot baby food

START WITH 3 medium carrots or 1½ cups baby carrots

1. prep

Wash and peel the carrots. Cut off the stems and tip, then cut in half cross-wise. Chop into 1-inch pieces.

2. cook

There are several options for cooking carrots.

MICROWAVE

cook time: 3 minutes

Place carrots in a microwave-safe bowl with 1 tablespoon of water. Cover and cook for 3–6 minutes, or until tender.

STEAM

cook time: 7 minutes

Set up a steamer basket in a medium pot. Add enough water to reach just below the basket. Then bring to a boil. Cover and steam the carrots until tender (about 7 minutes).

BOIL

cook time: 7 minutes

Bring a medium pot to a boil. Add carrots and cook for 7–10 minutes, or until tender. Drain the carrots in a colander.

SAUTÉ

cook time: 10 minutes

Heat 1 tablespoon of butter in a sauté pan over medium heat. Add the carrots cover and cook for 10–15 minutes, or until tender.

ROAST

cook time: 25 minutes

Heat oven to 400°F. Line a sheet pan with aluminum foil and spray with cooking spray. Spread the carrots on top. Roast for 25 minutes, or until tender. Shake the roasting pan halfway through to rotate the carrots.

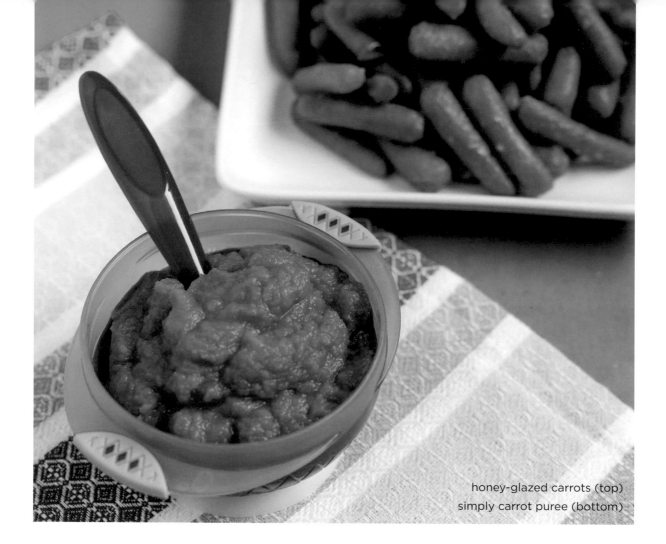

honey-glazed carrots (top)
simply carrot puree (bottom)

3. add mix-ins & serve

Serve simple or with tasty mix-ins. Puree, mash, or dice according to your baby's stage.

simply carrot puree

6 months +

MIX-INS

¾ cup breast milk, formula, or water

Transfer cooked carrots to a food processor with breast milk, formula, or water. Puree until smooth and soupy.

carrot-sweet potato puree

7 months +

MIX-INS

1 sweet potato

¾ cup breast milk, formula, or water

Wash the potato, then use a fork to poke holes all over. Place on a microwave-safe dish and microwave for 9 minutes, or until tender. Cut in half, and then scoop out the potato. Place the carrots and sweet potato in a food processor with breast milk, formula, or water and whirl until smooth.

carrot-apple puree

8 months +

MIX-INS

1 large apple

½ cup breast milk, formula, or water

Peel, quarter, and core the apple. Cook the apple until tender (3 minutes in the microwave, 12 minutes steamed, or 15 minutes baked at 375°F). Transfer the apples and cooked carrots to a food processor with the breast milk, formula, or water. Blend to create a smooth, thick puree.

carrots with lentils

9 months +

MIX-INS

¼ cup uncooked red lentils

½ cup breast milk, formula, or water

Rinse the lentils, removing any shriveled lentils or small rocks. Place 1 cup of water in a small saucepan, and add the lentils. Bring to a boil. Simmer for 30 minutes, or until tender. Drain the lentils, and then add them to the bowl of a food processor with the cooked carrots and breast milk, formula, or water. Pulse to create a coarse and chunky puree.

carrots and beef

10 months +

MIX-INS

¼ pound ground beef

Sauté the beef over medium-high heat in a skillet. Use a spatula to chop up the meat. Cook through. Drain any grease from the pan. Then place beef in a food processor with the cooked carrots. Puree until coarse and chunky.

carrot and pea medley

11 months +

MIX-INS

½ cup peas

Cook peas until tender (microwave for 2 minutes, steam or boil for 3 minutes). Place the carrots in a food processor and blitz once or twice to chop into bite-sized pieces. Mix together in a small bowl with the peas and serve as finger food.

carrots with turkey

12 months +

MIX-INS

1 small, skinless turkey breast

Cook the turkey until no longer pink (sauté for 5 minutes or bake for 15 minutes at 350°F). Dice the cooked carrots and turkey into bite-sized pieces, then scatter a few pieces onto baby's tray, adding more pieces as he eats them.

honey-glazed carrots

total time: 15 minutes

This easy, healthy side dish is awesome for a busy weeknight dinner, and delicious enough for holidays.

1 tablespoon butter

2 cups baby carrots

2 tablespoons honey

⅓ teaspoon ground ginger

Place the carrots in a sauté pan and cover with water. Bring to a boil, cover, and cook 7–10 minutes until tender. Drain and set aside.

Heat the butter in the sauté pan over medium heat. Add the carrots, honey, and ginger, and cook until the carrots are coated in a honey-butter glaze.

carrot-sweet potato mash

preparation time: 10 minutes

cook time: 20 minutes

1 large sweet potato, peeled and cut into ¾-inch cubes

1 cup baby carrots, or peeled whole carrots cut into 2-inch sticks

1 tablespoon brown sugar

2 tablespoons butter

2 tablespoons milk

Fill a medium pot with water and bring to a boil. Add the potatoes and cook for 5 minutes. Then add the carrots and cook for 10 more minutes, or until the potatoes and carrots are tender.

Drain the potatoes and carrots. Puree with a blender or immersion blender until smooth. Mix in the brown sugar, butter, and milk until just incorporated.

smooth carrot and lentil soup

preparation time: 5 minutes

cook time: 40 minutes

2 tablespoons olive oil

½ cup yellow onion, chopped

1½ cup red lentils, rinsed and picked

3 cups baby carrots

5 cups vegetable stock

crusty bread or naan for serving

Place the oil in a large pot, and heat over medium heat. Add the onions and sauté until soft, about 6 minutes.

Add the lentils, carrots, vegetable broth, and spices, and stir to combine. Bring to a boil, then reduce heat to low, cover and cook for 30 minutes until the lentils are soft.

Puree the soup with the milk in a blender or immersion blender until smooth and creamy. Season to taste with salt and pepper. Serve piping hot with crusty bread or naan.

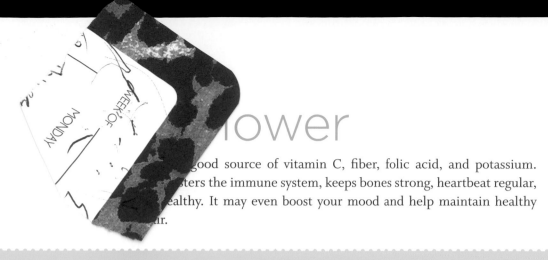

...ower

...good source of vitamin C, fiber, folic acid, and potassium. ...ters the immune system, keeps bones strong, heartbeat regular, ...ealthy. It may even boost your mood and help maintain healthy ...r.

cauliflower baby food

START WITH 2 cups fresh or frozen cauliflower florets and stems

1. prep

Take one head of cauliflower and cut off the end of the stalk. Chop the cauliflower into florets, cutting out and discarding any brown, wilted, or mushy stems or sprouts. Wash thoroughly.

2. cook

Cook frozen cauliflower as directed on the bag. If using fresh cauliflower, choose one of the following cooking methods.

MICROWAVE

cook time: 4 minutes

Place the cauliflower in a microwave-safe bowl with 1 tablespoon of water. Cover and cook until tender, about 4 minutes.

BOIL

cook time: 5 minutes

Bring a medium pot of water to boil. Add the cauliflower and cook until tender, about 5–8 minutes. Drain the cauliflower in a colander.

STEAM

cook time: 6 minutes

Set up a steamer basket in a medium pot and add enough water so it reaches just below the basket. Bring to a boil. Add the cauliflower, then cover and steam for 6–10 minutes, or until tender.

ROAST

cook time: 25 minutes

Preheat the oven to 400°F. Spread the cauliflower out on a sheet pan lined with parchment paper and roast for 25 minutes or until tender.

3. add mix-ins & serve

simply cauliflower puree

8 months +

MIX-INS

⅓ cup breast milk, formula or water

Transfer the cooked cauliflower to a food processor with breast milk, formula, or water, and whirl until smooth.

cauliflower-carrot puree

9 months +

MIX-INS

1 cup baby carrots, or peeled and chopped carrots

½ cup breast milk, formula, or water

Cook the carrots until tender (microwave for 3 minutes, steam or boil for 7 minutes, sauté with butter for 10 minutes, or roast for 25 minutes at 400°F). Transfer the cauliflower, carrots, and breast milk, formula, or water to a food processor and pulse to create a soft, lumpy puree.

creamy mashed cauliflower

10 months +

MIX-INS

2½ tablespoons cream cheese

1 tablespoon breast milk, formula, or water

Puree the cooked cauliflower, cream cheese, and breast milk, formula, or water in a food processor to create a soft, mashed consistency.

cauliflower and chicken

11 months +

MIX-INS

1 small, skinless chicken breast

Cook the chicken until no longer pink (sauté for 10 minutes, poach for 10 minutes, grill for 12 minutes, or bake for 15 minutes at 375°F). Finely dice ⅓ cup cauliflower and ⅓ cup chicken. Serve a few pieces at a time as finger food.

cauliflower and zucchini

12 months +

MIX-INS

⅓ cup diced zucchini, cooked

Microwave or sauté the zucchini until tender. Finely dice the cauliflower and zucchini into bite-sized pieces, and mix together in a bowl and serve as finger food.

parmesan roasted cauliflower

preparation time: 5 minutes

cook time: 35 minutes

3 cups cauliflower florets

2 tablespoons olive oil

1 teaspoon Italian seasoning

½ cup Parmesan cheese

Preheat the oven to 450°F. Cover a baking sheet with aluminum foil.

Spread the florets onto the baking sheet in a single layer. Then drizzle with oil and sprinkle with herbs, salt, and pepper.

Roast for 20 minutes, tossing halfway through. Sprinkle with Parmesan, then roast until the cauliflower is tender, 5 minutes longer.

mashed cauliflower with chives

total time: 25 minutes

1 head cauliflower, cut into florets

4 garlic cloves

⅜ cup cream cheese

2 tablespoons chives, diced

Bring a large pot of water to boil. Add the cauliflower and garlic and cook until tender (about 10 minutes). Drain in a colander.

Place the cauliflower and garlic back in the pot, and then add the cream cheese. Use a stick blender to puree until smooth. Season to taste with salt and pepper, and top with chives.

cauliflower mac'n cheese

preparation time: 10 minutes

cook time: 15 minutes

1 head cauliflower, cut into florets

3 tablespoons butter

1 cup onion, diced

2 tablespoons flour

2 cups milk

1½ cups swiss cheese

½ cup cheddar cheese

¼ teaspoon cayenne

Bring a large pot of water to a boil. Add cauliflower florets and cook until al dente, about 5 minutes. Drain and set aside.

To make the cheese sauce, add the butter and onion to a skillet, and cook until the onion is soft, about 6 minutes. Stir in the flour, coating the onion. Briefly remove from the burner and stir in the milk.

With the skillet back on the heat, cook on medium until thickened. Make sure the milk doesn't boil. Whisk in more flour to thicken if needed. Remove from the heat, and stir in the cheese and cayenne until combined. Season with salt and pepper.

Add the cauliflower to the cheese sauce, and stir to coat. Serve as a main dish or side.

green peas

Peas are a type of legume and a vitamin powerhouse. They have supersize servings of fiber and vitamins C and K, and are an excellent source of vegetable protein with about 8 grams per cup. Peas are a great food for babies because they help build strong bones, muscles, and healthy nerves. In adults, they may fight off symptoms of depression.

pea baby food

START WITH 1 cup of fresh or frozen peas

1. prep

If using fresh peas, tear off the top of one pea pod, then pull on the string to open it. Pop the peas out with your fingers, and then wash them in a colander. (This will take some time.)

2. cook

Cook frozen peas as directed on the bag. If using fresh peas, choose from the following cooking methods.

MICROWAVE

cook time: 2 minutes

Place peas in a microwave-safe bowl with 1 tablespoon of water. Cover and microwave on high until tender, about 2 minutes.

STEAM

cook time: 2 minutes

Put a steamer basket in a saucepan and fill with water to just below the basket. Bring the water to a boil. Add the peas to the basket, and then cover and cook for 2 minutes.

BOIL

cook time: 3 minutes

Add peas to a saucepan and just with water (use as little water as you can). Bring to a boil, cooking about 3 minutes. Drain the peas in a colander.

3. add mix-ins & serve

simply pea puree

9 months +

MIX-INS

1 tablespoon breast milk, formula, or water

Puree the peas and breast milk, formula, or water in a food processor to form a soft mashed puree with tiny lumps.

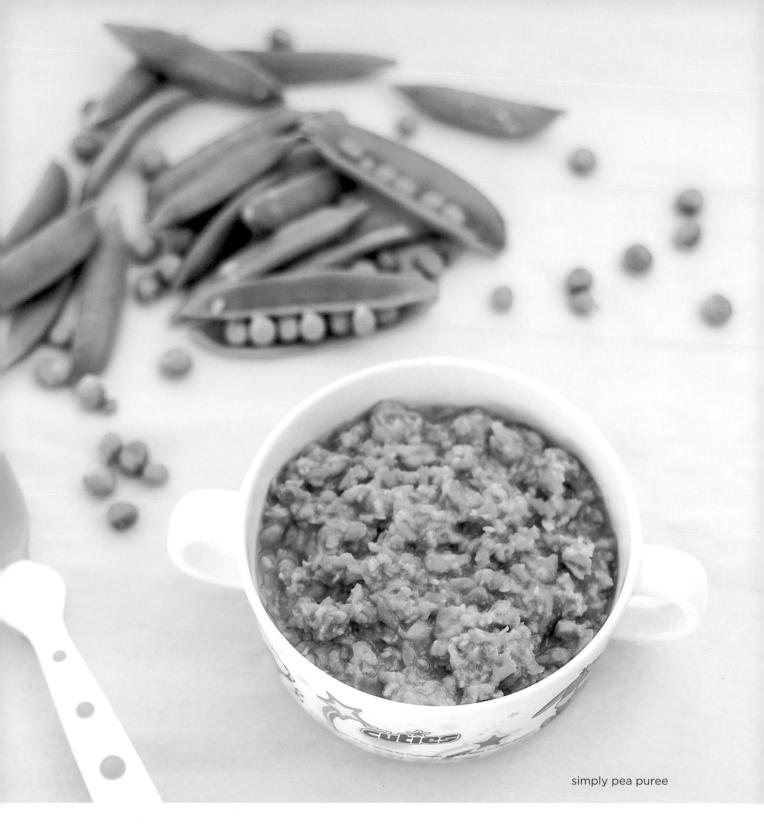

simply pea puree

green peas

pea-asparagus puree

10 months +

MIX-INS

6 asparagus, trimmed

3 tablespoons breast milk, formula, or water

Cook asparagus until tender (microwave for 2 minutes, boil for 3 minutes, steam for 4 minutes or roast for 15 minutes at 400°F). Place the peas, asparagus, and breast milk, formula, or water in a blender and puree until smooth.

pea poppers

11 months +

Serve the peas whole as finger food. Let baby have fun popping the peas in his mouth, or squishing them with his fingers.

tuna and pea pasta

12 months +

MIX-INS

¼ cup cooked pasta

½ tablespoon canned tuna, drained

This recipe is meant to be paired with the adult recipe that follows. Mix ¼ cup peas (reserving the rest for another meal), pasta, and tuna together in a small bowl until combined.

mama recipes

smashed peas

total time: 10 minutes

This British side dish is also known as mushy peas and is traditionally served with fish and chips, meat roasts, savory pies, and more. It's simple to make and full of flavor, making it a fantastic way to eat peas.

1½ cups frozen peas

1½ tablespoons butter

1 tablespoon milk

Place the peas in a medium saucepan and cover with water. Boil and cook for 2 minutes. Then drain the water.

Melt the butter in the saucepan, and then add the peas back into the pan. Use a potato masher to smash the peas to a mix of mashed and semi-solid. Season generously with salt and pepper. Then stir in the milk until combined.

vegetables

mushroom and pea stroganoff

preparation time: 10 minutes

cook time: 25 minutes

4 cups dried egg noodles

4 tablespoons butter

3 garlic cloves, minced

¼ cup onion, thinly sliced

2 ½ cups sliced cremini or white mushrooms

1 cup frozen peas, thawed

1 tablespoon cornstarch

½ cup vegetable stock

¼ cup white wine

½ cup sour cream

Bring a large pot of salted water to a boil. Add the egg noodles and cook 6–8 minutes, or until tender.

Meanwhile, heat a skillet over medium heat. Then add butter, garlic, onion, mushrooms, and peas. Cook until the onions are soft and the mushrooms and peas are tender, about 5 minutes.

Add the cornstarch to the pan, stirring to coat the vegetables. Add the wine and stock, and then heat on medium-high until boiling. Cook for about 5 minutes to thicken. Turn the burner off. Stir in the sour cream until combined. Season well with salt and pepper.

Serve the veggie stroganoff over egg noodles.

green pea soup

preparation time: 5 minutes

cook time: 15 minutes

2 tablespoons butter

½ white onion, diced

3 cups frozen peas

2 cups chicken stock

3 tablespoons milk

crusty baguette bread

In a large pot, melt the butter over medium heat. Then add the onion. Sauté until soft, about 5 minutes.

Add frozen peas and stock to the pot, bring to a boil, and then reduce the heat to low. Cover and simmer until the peas are tender (about 10 minutes).

Add the milk and puree with an immersion or traditional blender until smooth and creamy. Pour into serving bowls and top with salt and pepper. Serve with a big piece of crusty bread for dipping.

tuna pasta salad with peas

total time: 20 minutes

Growing up, my mom would always make this dish for BBQs or family gatherings, and it was always a hit. Now that I'm a mama, I like to make it ahead for an easy lunch.

2½ cups tri-color rotini pasta

1 cup frozen peas

1 can flaked tuna, drained

⅓ cup mayonnaise

Bring a large pot of salted water to a boil.

Add the rotini pasta and cook for 9 minutes. When you have 2 minutes left, add the peas. Then drain in a colander.

Rinse the pasta and peas with cold water to cool. Toss to remove excess water.

Pour the pasta and peas into a large bowl and stir in the tuna and mayonnaise. Season generously with salt and pepper. Keep covered in the refrigerator until serving.

potatoes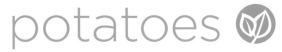

These root vegetables are packed with antioxidants, fiber, potassium, and vitamin C. They help fight free radicals (which can damage cells and are are associated with causing diseases) in the body and maintain healthy blood pressure and blood sugar.

Additionally, sweet potatoes are rich in beta-carotene, promoting healthy eyes, skin, and immune systems. Beta-carotene, which changes to vitamin A in the body, may also reduce the risk of heart disease and cancer.

russet and sweet potato baby food

START WITH 1 large russet or sweet potato

1. prep

Scrub the potato under cold water.

2. cook

Choose from the following cooking methods.

MICROWAVE

cook time: 9 minutes

Use a fork to pierce all over the skin of the potato. Place the potato on a microwave-safe dish and cook for 4 minutes. Turn over, then continue cooking until tender, about 5 more minutes. Use a spoon to scoop out the potato, discarding the skin.

BOIL

cook time: 10 minutes

Peel the potato, then rinse. Chop into large chunks, then place in a saucepan and cover with water. Bring to a boil. Cook until tender, about 5–15 minutes. Drain in a colander.

ROAST

cook time: 30 minutes

Preheat the oven to 425°F. Peel, then chop the potato into 1-inch chunks and toss with olive oil. Place the potatoes in a single layer on a baking sheet lined with aluminum foil. Roast until the potatoes are tender, flipping halfway through, about 30 minutes.

BAKE

cook time: 60 minutes

Preheat the oven to 350°F. Pierce the skin of the potato several times with a fork. Place the potato on the middle rack in the oven and cook for 60 minutes, or until tender. Cut the potato in half and use a spoon to scoop out the inside. Discard the skin.

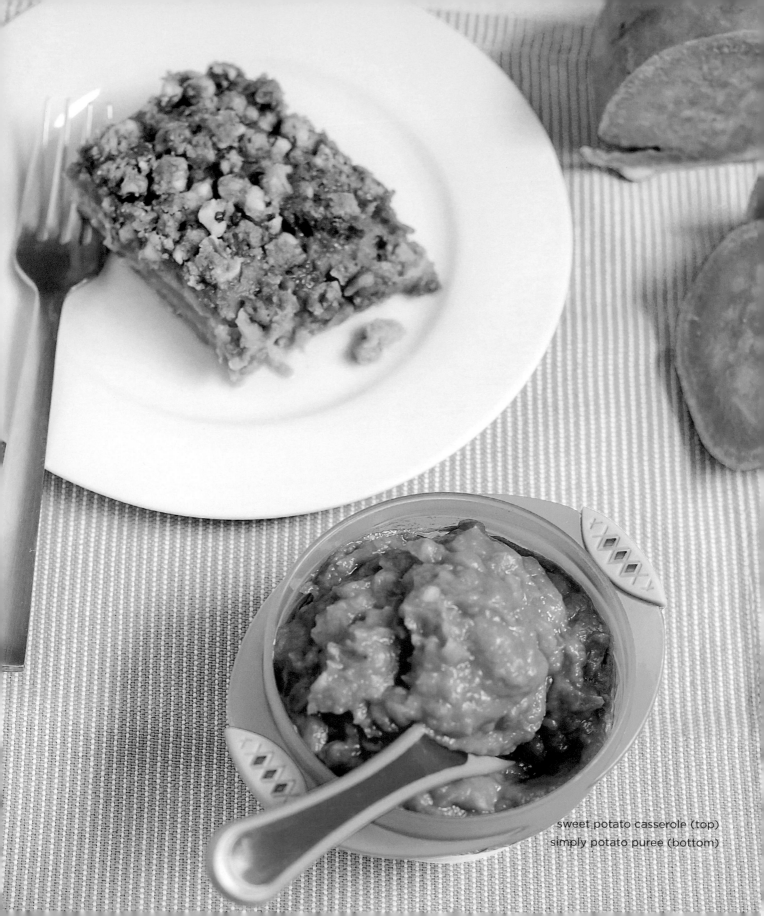

sweet potato casserole (top)
simply potato puree (bottom)

3. add mix-ins & serve

Serve on its own or with tasty mix-ins. Pureeing potatoes can overwork the potatoes and make them starchy and gluey. To avoid this, mash with a potato masher, food mill, or ricer for smoother potatoes.

simply potato puree

6–9 months + for sweet potatoes
9 months + for russet potatoes

MIX-INS

½ **cup breast milk, formula, or water**

Place the potato in a mixing bowl with the breast milk, formula, or water. Mash until smooth for 6–8 months; or thick with tiny lumps for 9+ months.

sweet potato, banana, and spinach puree

10 months +

MIX-INS

¾ **cup fresh spinach**

½ **banana**

½ **cup breast milk, formula, or water**

Wash the spinach and cook until wilted (microwave for 2 minutes, steam or sauté 2–5 minutes, or boil for 3–5 minutes). Meanwhile, mash the potato so that it's mostly smooth with a few lumps. Place the spinach, banana, and breast milk, formula, or water in the bowl of a food processor. Puree until smooth, and then mash into the potato.

turnip and russet mashed potatoes

11 months +

MIX-INS

1 **turnip**

½ **cup breast milk, formula, or water**

Peel, then chop the turnips, cutting away the greens. Cook the turnips until tender (microwave for 5 minutes, steam for 12 minutes, boil for 15 minutes, or roast for 25 minutes at 425°F). Mash the potatoes, turnips, and breast milk, formula, or water to form a soft, lumpy puree.

potato and cheese

12 months +

MIX-INS

2 **tablespoons cheddar or Monterey jack cheese**

Dice the potato into bite-sized pieces. Place ½ cup of potato in a small bowl and top with cheese. Serve as finger food.

mixed roasted potatoes

preparation time: 10 minutes
cook time: 10–30 minutes

1 medium russet potato

1 medium sweet potato

1 tablespoon olive oil

1 tablespoon Italian seasoning

There are two ways to cook these potatoes. Microwaving is the quickest and easiest method, but oven roasting develops more flavor and texture. If cooking in the oven, preheat to 425°F.

Wash the potatoes and cut into 1½-inch cubes. In a large bowl, toss them in olive oil and Italian seasoning until completely coated. Season with salt and pepper.

Microwave version: Pour the potatoes into a large microwave-safe dish. Microwave for 8–10 minutes, or until tender, tossing twice to rearrange the potatoes in the bowl.

Oven version: Cover a baking sheet with aluminum foil and place the potatoes in a single layer on the baking sheet. Roast for 30 minutes, or until the potatoes are tender and crispy, stirring halfway through.

chili and cheese baked potato

total time: 15 minutes

This hearty baked potato whips up in just 15 minutes, making it a quick lunch or dinner option.

2 russet potatoes, washed

1 (15-ounce) can of chili

2 tablespoons butter

2 cups shredded cheddar or Monterey jack cheese

½ cup sour cream

Prick the potatoes all over with a fork. Place on a sturdy microwave-safe dish and microwave for 10–12 minutes (depending on the size of the potatoes), flipping halfway through. Meanwhile, heat the chili in a small saucepan until hot.

Cut the potatoes in half lengthwise, and mash the insides with butter, forming little bowls out of the potato halves. Top with chili, cheese, and sour cream.

sweet potato casserole

preparation time: 20 minutes

cook time: 30 minutes

leftovers: 3 sides

This is no ordinary sweet potato casserole. It's lighter than most and doesn't overload on sweetness. Make this as a side for weeknight dinner (you'll love the leftovers!), or bring it to a holiday party to share with family and friends. It goes well with roasted chicken, turkey, and ham.

2 medium sweet potatoes

2 eggs, beaten

¾ cup granulated sugar

½ cup milk

1 teaspoon vanilla extract

½ teaspoon salt

3 tablespoons butter, melted

topping

½ cup brown sugar

4 tablespoons butter, melted

½ cup flour

¾ cup walnuts

Preheat the oven to 400°F, then grease an 8 × 8 inch baking dish. Pierce the potatoes all over with a fork, and microwave until cooked, about 8–15 minutes, flipping halfway through.

Meanwhile, whisk together the eggs, sugar, milk, vanilla, and salt. In a separate bowl, make the topping. Use a spoon to combine the brown sugar, butter, flour, and walnuts.

Scoop the flesh from the potatoes into a medium bowl. Then stir in the melted butter. Add the egg mixture, and stir until combined. It will look very liquidy, but this will make for a light and fluffy casserole.

Pour the sweet potato mixture into the prepared baking dish and add topping. Bake for 25 minutes, or until the potatoes are bubbling and the top is browned and crispy.

baked sweet potato fries

preparation time: 5 minutes

cook time: 20 minutes

1 sweet potato

1 tablespoon olive oil

⅛ teaspoon paprika

Preheat the oven to 450°F and line a baking sheet with parchment paper. Slice the potatoes into ½-inch fries.

In a medium bowl, toss the potatoes with olive oil, paprika, and salt and pepper.

Spread the potatoes in a single layer on the prepared baking sheet. Cook for 10 minutes, and then flip the fries and bake for another 10 minutes until golden brown and crispy.

pumpkins

This fall favorite is an excellent source of fiber and iron, as well as a variety of other vitamins and minerals. Its hearty supply of beta-carotene delivers over 200% of the recommended daily intake of vitamin A, and its fiber slows digestion to keep you feeling fuller, longer. The nutrients in pumpkin also help boost mood and immune system function, helping keep eyesight sharp, and skin wrinkle-free. It may also ward off certain cancers and maintain a healthy heart.

pumpkin baby food

START WITH 1 (4–6 pound) baking pumpkin or 2 cups fresh or frozen cubed pumpkin

1. prep

Wash the pumpkin, being sure to remove any dirt or debris. Remove the stem. Then, using a large knife, cut the pumpkin in half from top to bottom. Scoop out the seeds and stringy pulp with a large spoon. (Save the seeds if you are planning to eat them.)

If pumpkins aren't in season, you can use frozen, cubed pumpkin for baby food recipes or 100% canned pumpkin for adult recipes.

2. cook

Choose your cooking method based on whether you have pumpkin halves or cubes.

MICROWAVE

cook time: 5-15 minutes

If using halves, place pumpkin cut-side down in a microwave-safe dish with a splash of water. Cover and cook until tender, about 15 minutes. Scoop out 1¼ cups of soft pumpkin.

If using cubes, place in a microwave-safe dish with a splash of water and cook for 5–10 minutes, or until tender.

STEAM

cook time: 12 minutes

This method is best using pumpkin cubes. Set up a steamer basket in a medium pot, and add enough water to reach just below the basket. Bring the water to a boil. Add the pumpkin and cover and steam until tender, about 12 minutes.

BOIL

cook time: 10 minutes

This method is also best using pumpkin cubes. Bring a medium pot of water to a boil. Add the pumpkin and cook for 10–15 minutes, or until tender.

vegetables

ROAST

cook time: 30 minutes

If using pumpkin halves, preheat oven to 400°F. Place the pumpkin halves flesh-side down on a baking sheet lined with aluminum foil and spray with cooking spray. Roast for 30 minutes or until fork-tender. Scoop out 1¼ cups of soft pumpkin.

If using pumpkin cubes, place on a baking sheet and toss with olive oil. Roast for 30 minutes, or until tender.

3. add mix-ins & serve

Serve on its own or with tasty mix-ins. Puree, mash, or dice according to your baby's stage.

simply pumpkin puree

7 months +

MIX-INS

¼ cup breast milk, formula, or water

Transfer the cooked pumpkin to a food processor and puree with breast milk, formula, or water to form a smooth and soupy puree.

pumpkin-banana puree

8 months +

MIX-INS

1 banana, peeled

¼ cup breast milk, formula, or water

Puree the pumpkin, banana, and breast milk, formula, or water in a food processor until smooth.

apple-pumpkin puree

9 months +

MIX-INS

1 apple

¼ cup breast milk, formula, or water

Peel the apple and chop into small chunks. Cook until soft (microwave for 3–4 minutes, boil for 10 minutes, steam or bake for 15 minutes at 375°F). Transfer the apple and pumpkin to a food processor and whirl to form a soft, mashed puree without any lumps.

creamy chicken and pumpkin

10 months +

MIX-INS

1 small chicken breast (about ½ cup diced chicken)

⅓ cup breast milk or formula

Cook the chicken until it is cooked through (sauté for 10 minutes, grill for 12 minutes, poach for 10 minutes, or bake for 15 minutes at 375°F). Chop the chicken and transfer to a food processor with the pumpkin and breast milk or formula. Whirl to form a soft, lumpy puree.

pumpkin oats

11 months +

MIX-INS

½ cup old-fashioned rolled oats

1 tablespoon breast milk or formula

Bring 1 cup of water to a boil in a small saucepan. Add oats and cook for 5 minutes. Strain any excess water using a colander. Transfer the oatmeal, pumpkin, and breast milk or formula into a blender and pulse 2–3 times to make a chunky puree.

baby pumpkin pasta

12 months +

MIX-INS

¼ cup cooked elbow pasta

1 tablespoon shredded mozzarella cheese

This recipe is meant to be paired with the adult version that follows. Finely dice the pumpkin. Then in a small bowl, mix the pasta, cheese, and ⅛ cup of pumpkin (reserve the rest for another meal) until combined.

mama recipes

baked chocolate chip pumpkin oatmeal

preparation: 10 minutes

cook time: 25 minutes

leftovers: 2 meals

This oatmeal is hearty with a gentle sweetness. It cooks to a firm texture, a nice change from soft oatmeal. Prepare it the night before by mixing all of the dry ingredients together and all of the wet ingredients together in separate bowls and refrigerate. In the morning, combine and bake.

dry ingredients

2 cups rolled oats

1 teaspoon baking powder

¼ cup + 2 tablespoons brown sugar

1½ teaspoon pumpkin pie spice

½ cup semi-sweet chocolate chips

wet ingredients

1 cup pumpkin puree

1 egg, beaten

1 cup milk

2 tablespoons melted butter

1 teaspoons vanilla extract

Preheat the oven to 400°F. Combine all of the dry ingredients in a medium bowl. In a separate bowl, combine the wet ingredients. Stir the wet ingredients into the dry ingredients.

Pour into a buttered 8 × 8 baking dish or unbuttered Dutch oven. Bake for 20 minutes. Then place under a broiler for 2–3 minutes to crisp the top.

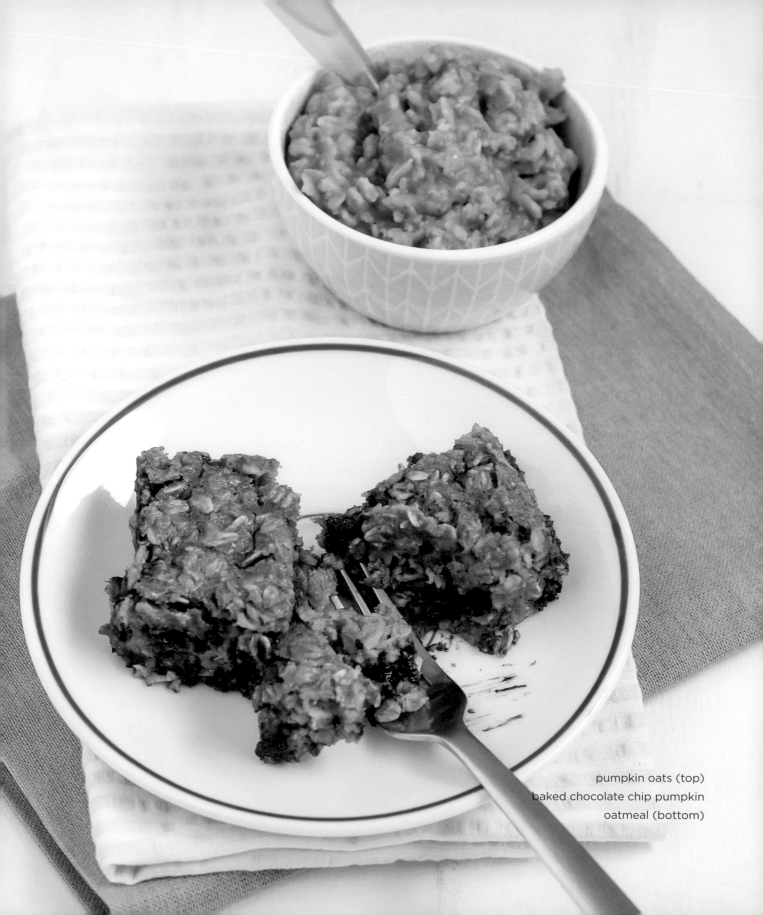

pumpkin oats (top)
baked chocolate chip pumpkin
oatmeal (bottom)

pumpkin tortellini alfredo

preparation time: 5 minutes

cook time: 10 minutes

Back when it was just my husband and me, we used to make almost everything from scratch, including Alfredo sauce. Now with baby, I usually choose jarred sauces—so much easier! I've also found that by adding a few ingredients, you can transform a plain store-bought sauce into something fresh and flavorful.

2 cups cheese tortellini

1 cup good-quality Alfredo sauce

½ cup pumpkin puree

¼ teaspoon Italian seasoning

⅛ teaspoon nutmeg

¼ cup Parmesan cheese

1 tablespoon fresh basil, cut into strips

Cook the tortellini as directed on the box. After it's cooked, drain the water and pour the tortellini back in the pot.

While the tortellini is cooking, combine the Alfredo sauce, pumpkin puree, Italian seasoning, and nutmeg in a medium saucepan. Heat on medium-low until warm, and then pour the sauce over the tortellini and stir to coat. Divide between two bowls and serve sprinkled with Parmesan cheese and basil.

slow-cooker spinach and pumpkin pasta

preparation time: 10 minutes

slow-cook time: 4 hours

leftovers: 2 meals

1¼ cups ricotta

1½ cups shredded mozzarella cheese

½ cup Parmesan cheese

½ teaspoon salt

1¾ cups marinara sauce

2¾ cups uncooked elbow pasta or ziti

2 cups fresh or frozen cubed pumpkin

2 cups fresh spinach

In a medium bowl, combine the ricotta, ½ cup of mozzarella cheese, Parmesan cheese, and salt.

Spray the inside of the slower cooker with cooking spray. Pour in half the sauce, ½ cup water, and all of the pasta. Stir together to moisten the pasta—this helps the pasta cook. Then top with pumpkin and spinach. Spoon the cheese mixture over the spinach and top with remaining sauce.

Cover and cook on low for 4–5 hours or until the pasta is tender. Sprinkle with the remaining mozzarella cheese, and then cover and cook for another 10 minutes to melt the cheese.

spinach

This leafy green is packed with vitamins, antioxidants, and minerals. Spinach is an excellent source of folic acid, iron, and calcium in particular. It's also a good source of plant-based omega-3s. Spinach is great for your muscles (Popeye was right!), bones, and teeth. It promotes healthy growth in children, can help restore energy (for those times you're feeling sluggish), and may even ward off symptoms of depression and PMS.

Spinach contains nitrates. Though it's a super nutritious ingredient and safe for baby to eat after 10 months, limit meals with spinach to only a few feedings a week.

spinach baby food

START WITH 1 (1 pound) package fresh spinach or 1 (10-ounce) bag frozen spinach

1. prep

If using fresh spinach, empty it into a large bowl. Remove any brown, wilted, or deteriorated leaves. Clean the spinach well—even if it's pre-washed—to help rinse off any E. coli organisms that are sometimes present in fresh spinach. For an extra good clean, soak the spinach in a bath of 3 cups white vinegar to 1 cup of water for 2–5 minutes. Then place it in a colander over the sink. Drain and rinse thoroughly with cold water.

2. cook

If using frozen spinach, cook as directed on the bag, squeezing out any excess water. If using fresh spinach, choose from the following cooking methods.

MICROWAVE

cook time: 2 minutes

Place spinach in a large microwave-safe baking dish with a splash of water. Cover and microwave until tender, about 2–4 minutes.

SAUTÉ

cook time: 3 minutes

Heat a large skillet over medium heat. Melt 1 tablespoon butter or olive oil in the pan, and then add the spinach. Cook, stirring about 3–5 minutes until the spinach is wilted.

BOIL

cook time: 3 minutes

Fill a large pot with water and bring to a boil over medium-high heat. Add the spinach and then cook until tender, about 3–5 minutes. Pour the spinach into a colander over the sink and drain the water.

STEAM

cook time: 4 minutes

Set up a steamer basket in a pot and add enough water so it reaches just below the basket. Bring to a boil. Add the spinach to the basket. (It may take a couple batches depending on the size of your pot and basket.) Cover and steam until tender, about 4–6 minutes.

3. add mix-ins & serve

Serve on its own or with tasty mix-ins.

simply spinach puree

10 months +

MIX-INS

½ tablespoon breast milk, formula, or water

Place the spinach and breast milk, formula, or water in a food processor and whirl to create a chunky puree.

spinach apple banana

11 months +

MIX-INS

1 apple

1 banana, peeled

2 tablespoons breast milk, formula, or water

Peel the apple. Then cut it in half and remove the core and seeds. Cook until tender (microwave for 3–4 minutes, boil for 10 minutes, steam for 12 minutes, or bake for 15 minutes at 375°F). Place the spinach, apple, banana, and breast milk, formula, or water in a food processor to make a chunky puree.

chopped egg yolk and spinach

12 months +

MIX-INS

4 hard-boiled eggs, shelled

Remove the egg yolk and finely dice with ½ cup of spinach. Stir the spinach and egg yolks together in a small bowl.

simple sautéed spinach

preparation time: 5 minutes

cook time: 5 minutes

1 tablespoon olive oil

1 (10-ounce) package fresh spinach, washed thoroughly

2 garlic cloves, diced

Heat the olive oil in a large skillet over medium heat. Add the spinach and garlic. Cook, stirring occasionally, until the spinach is wilted, about 3–5 minutes. Season with salt and pepper.

creamed spinach

preparation time: 10 minutes

cook time: 10 minutes

2 tablespoons olive oil

2 garlic cloves, minced

½ cup white onion, diced

7 cups fresh spinach, washed thoroughly

⅓ cup milk

2 tablespoons butter

3 tablespoons all-purpose flour

⅛ teaspoon nutmeg

¼ cup grated Parmesan cheese

In a large saucepan, heat the oil over medium-low heat. Add the garlic and onion, and cook until soft. Keep an eye on the garlic to make sure it doesn't burn. Reduce the heat if it starts to brown.

Whisk in the flour. Then stir in the milk, butter, and nutmeg. Cook until thickened, about 5 minutes. Stir in the spinach, cooking until spinach is wilted, about 7 minutes. Season generously with salt and pepper. Then remove from the heat and stir in the cheese until combined.

spinach and egg breakfast sandwich

total time: 20 minutes

4 bacon slices

1 (10-ounce) package of frozen spinach

2 eggs

2 tablespoons butter

2 English muffins

Arrange the bacon side-by-side on a microwave-safe dish. Then cover with a paper towel and microwave for 3–5 minutes, or until crispy. Blot excess grease with paper towels.

Cook the spinach according to the package instructions.

Meanwhile, cook the eggs. Use an egg cooker or pan-fry to your liking. I recommend poached or over easy.

Toast and butter the English muffins and place on plates. Make your sandwiches by placing two pieces of bacon, one egg, and half the spinach on each bottom muffin. Cover with the muffin tops.

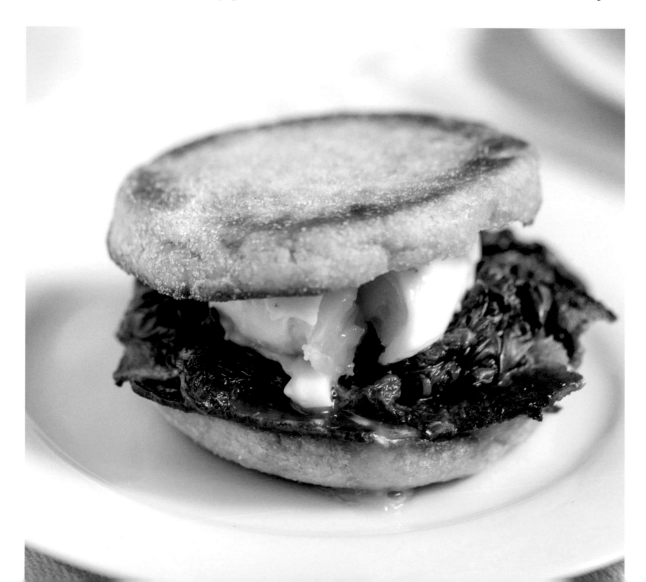

acorn and butternut squash

Though technically a fruit, winter squash is often used like a vegetable. It offers supersized servings of beta-carotene and vitamin C. It's also a great source of potassium and fiber. And since you digest winter squash slowly, it helps you feel full longer. It may also help fend off breast cancer, heal cuts and wounds, and keep teeth and gums healthy.

Winter squash is particularly helpful in the development of babies' lungs.

The hardest thing about squash is cutting it up. Sometimes you can find it already peeled and cut in the grocery store. Just check the prepared produce section. Look through the expiration dates to pick out the freshest one. Another handy shortcut is to use frozen, cubed squash; just follow the instructions on the bag for cooking.

Squash contains nitrates. Though it makes great baby food, and is safe for baby to eat after 7 months, limit meals with squash to only a few feedings a week.

acorn and butternut squash baby food

START WITH 1 acorn or butternut squash or 1¼ cups of chopped squash.

1. prep

Wash the outside of the squash. Use a large knife to cut it in half from top to bottom, and then scrape out the seeds and any remaining strings. Peel and cut into cubes if desired.

2. cook

Choose your cooking method based on whether you have squash halves or cubes.

MICROWAVE

cook time: 5-15 minutes

If using cubed squash, place in a microwave-safe dish with a splash of water, and cover and cook until tender, about 5–10 minutes.

If using squash halves, place facedown in a microwave-safe dish, and then add about a ½-inch of water. Microwave for 15 minutes. Scoop out 1 cup of squash.

STEAM

cook time: 12 minutes

This method works best with squash cubes. Set up a steamer basket in a medium pot, and then add enough water so it reaches just below the basket. Bring to a boil. Cover and steam the squash until tender, about 12 minutes.

BOIL

cook time: 13 minutes

This method works best with squash cubes. Bring a medium pot of water to a boil, and then add the squash and cook for 13 minutes, or until tender.

ROAST

cook time: 30 minutes

If using squash halves, preheat oven to 400°F. Place the squash halves facedown on a baking sheet lined with aluminum foil and sprayed with cooking spray. Roast until the squash is tender, about 30 minutes. Scoop out 1 cup of soft squash.

3. add mix-ins & serve

Serve on its own or with tasty mix-ins. Puree, mash, or dice according to your baby's stage.

simply winter squash puree

7 months +

MIX-INS

¼ cup breast milk, formula, or water

Puree cooked squash in a food processor with breast milk, formula, or water until smooth and soupy.

squash and brown rice cereal

8 months +

MIX-INS

¼ cup ground brown rice

¼ cup breast milk, formula, or water

Boil 1 cup of water in a small saucepan. Slowly pour in the rice cereal, whisking constantly for about a minute to prevent clumping. Cook the rice cereal for 15 minutes, stirring occasionally. Meanwhile, puree the squash until smooth. Stir the squash puree and breast milk, formula, or water into the rice cereal until combined.

winter squash and sweet potato puree

9 months +

MIX-INS

1 small sweet potato (about ½ cup)

½ cup breast milk, formula, or water

Scrub the potato. Then pierce the skin several times with a fork. Cook the potato in the microwave for 9 minutes, or bake for 60 minutes at 350°F. Cut in half and scoop the potato into a food processor. Puree the sweet potato, squash, and breast milk, formula, or water to create a soft puree with tiny lumps.

squash, apple, and pork

10 months +

MIX-INS

1 apple

1 thin pork chop, fat trimmed off

½ cup breast milk, formula, or water

Peel the apple and finely dice. Heat a tablespoon of oil in a medium skillet. Add the pork chops. Brown one side, then flip. Add the apples, and continue cooking until the pork is well-done, about 8 minutes total. Cut the pork in half. Place in a blender with the squash and apple, and breast milk, formula, or water. Whirl to form a lumpy puree.

squash, pear, and kale

11 months +

MIX-INS

½ pear

1 cup fresh kale, de-stemmed

Peel the pear, then cut in half and remove the core. Cook the pear and kale together until tender (microwave for 2 minutes, steam for 5 minutes, or sauté for 6 minutes). Place the pear, squash, and kale in a food processor and blitz to form a chunky puree.

buttery squash bites

12 months +

MIX-IN

¼ tablespoon unsalted butter

Dice a few cubes of squash into bite-sized pieces. Melt the butter in the microwave, and then drizzle over the squash. Let cool to room temperature. Serve as finger food.

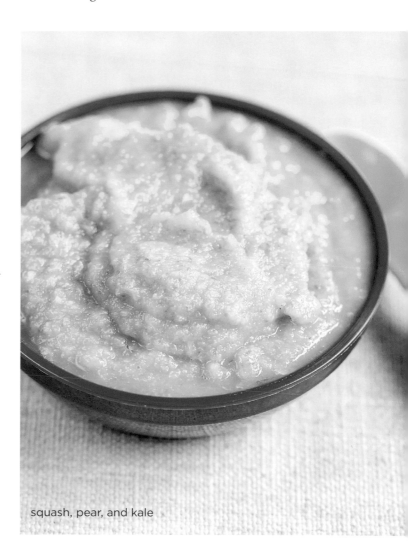

squash, pear, and kale

acorn and butternut squash

cinnamon and honey roasted squash

preparation time: 15 minutes

cook time: 45 minutes

1 acorn or butternut squash

2 tablespoons butter, diced

¼ teaspoon cinnamon

⅛ cup honey

Heat the oven to 400°F. Meanwhile, cut the squash in half lengthwise and scoop out the seeds and any remaining strings.

Place the squash halves cut-side up in a baking dish. Arrange the butter cubes in the center and on the ridges of the squash. Sprinkle with cinnamon and drizzle with honey. Season with salt and pepper.

Roast until tender, usually 45 minutes to an hour, depending on the size of the squash.

microwaved maple squash

total time: 10 minutes

4 cups fresh or frozen winter squash, peeled and cubed

2 tablespoons butter

1 tablespoon maple syrup

½ teaspoon cinnamon

2 tablespoons milk

Place the squash cubes and ⅛ cup water in a large microwave-safe bowl. Cover with a paper towel and microwave for 5 minutes, or until tender.

Pour out the water from the bottom of the bowl, then put the squash, butter, maple syrup, cinnamon and milk in a blender and puree until smooth.

slow cooker squash and apples

preparation time: 15 minutes

slow cook time: 3 hours

1 pound fresh winter squash, peeled and cubed

1 large apple, cubed

2 tablespoons butter, cut into pieces

⅛ cup brown sugar

¼ teaspoon pumpkin pie spice

Spray the slow cooker with cooking spray, then add the squash and apples. Top with butter pieces, then sprinkle with sugar and pumpkin pie spice. Cover and cook on high for 3 hours.

zucchini and summer squash

Zucchini and yellow summer squash offer hearty doses of vitamin C, potassium, and fiber, and promote healthy skin, hair, and teeth. They also strengthen the immune system, help prevent constipation and kidney stones, and promote healthy blood pressure.

Zucchini and yellow squash both contain nitrates. Although many experts say it's safe to feed your baby foods with nitrates after six months, you may want to limit intake to small, infrequent portions during his first year.

zucchini and summer squash baby food

START WITH 3 cups sliced zucchini or summer squash

1. prep

Wash one or two zucchini or summer squash (depending on their size). Cut off both ends of the squash, then peel. If you have a large squash, cut it in half and remove the seeds with a spoon. (Seeds from small zucchini and summer squash are easily digested.) Then cut into thin slices.

2. cook

Choose cooking method from the following options.

MICROWAVE

cook time: 5 minutes

Place squash in a microwave-safe baking dish with 1 tablespoon of water. Cover and microwave until tender, about 5 minutes.

GRILL

cook time: 5 minutes

Heat the grill to 350°F. Spray a sheet of aluminum foil with cooking spray and place the squash slices in a pile in the center of the foil. Fold to seal shut. Place the foil packet on the grill grates, and cook until tender, about 5–10 minutes.

STEAM

cook time: 5 minutes

Set up a steamer basket in a medium pot and add water to just below the basket. Bring to a boil. Cover and steam the squash until tender, about 5 minutes.

SAUTÉ

cook time: 8 minutes

Heat 1 tablespoon of olive oil or butter in a non-stick skillet over medium-high heat. Sauté the squash until tender, about 8–10 minutes.

3. add mix-ins & serve

Serve simply or with tasty mix-ins. Puree or finely dice according to your baby's stage.

simply squash puree

7 months +

MIX-INS

1 tablespoon breast milk, formula, or water

Transfer the zucchini and breast milk, formula, or water to a food processor, and puree until smooth.

squash-carrot puree

8 months +

MIX-INS

1 cup baby carrots

1 tablespoons breast milk, formula, or water

Cook the carrots until tender (microwave for 3 minutes, steam or boil for 7 minutes, or roast for 25 minutes at 400°F). Place the squash, carrots, and breast milk, formula, or water in a food processor and whirl to form a smooth, thick puree.

squash, potato, and turkey

9 months +

MIX-INS

½ small potato, peeled and chopped

1 small turkey breast

½ cup breast milk, formula, or water

Cook the chopped potatoes until tender (microwave for 9 minutes, boil for 10 minutes, or roast for 30 minutes at 425°F). Cook the turkey breast (sauté for 5 minutes, broil for 10 minutes, or bake for 15–20 minutes at 350°F). Chop the turkey, then place in the food processor with the potato and squash, and breast milk, formula or water. Pulse to create a smooth puree with tiny lumps.

squash-pea puree

10 months +

MIX-INS

1 cup green peas

2 tablespoons breast milk, formula, or water

Cook the peas until tender, 2 minutes in the microwave or 3 minutes steamed or boiled. Place the squash, peas, and breast milk, formula, or water in a food processor, and pulse to make a chunky puree.

cheesy parmesan squash

11 months +

MIX-INS

½ tablespoon grated Parmesan

Finely dice ½ cup of squash. Then place in a bowl and top with cheese. Serve a few pieces at a time as finger food.

steak and zucchini

12 months +

MIX-INS

¼ cup cooked steak

This recipe is meant to be paired with the adult kabob recipe that follows. Remove 2 steak cubes from the skewer and test for doneness (steak should be well-done for baby). Place back on the grill if needed, and cook until no longer pink. Let the steak cool to the touch. Then break off small pieces or shred steak. Chop ¼ cup of zucchini into bite-sized pieces. Serve a few pieces of steak and zucchini at a time as finger food.

squash and mushroom packets

preparation time: 10 minutes

cook time: 20 minutes

1 zucchini or summer squash, sliced

¾ cup sliced white mushroom

⅓ cup white onion, sliced

1 garlic clove, minced

1 tablespoon olive oil

1 teaspoon Italian seasoning

There are two ways to cook this dish—on the grill (preheat grill to medium-high) or the oven (preheat oven to 375°F).

Combine all the ingredients in a bowl and season with salt and pepper. Place the veggies in the center of a sheet of foil, and then fold to make a closed square packet, sealing the edges.

Grill or bake for 20 minutes or until tender, flipping once.

parmesan roasted zucchini sticks

preparation: 5 minutes

cook time: 15 minutes

1 large zucchini

¼ cup grated Parmesan cheese

olive oil

Preheat oven to 350°F. Cut the zucchini in half down the middle, and then quarter. Spread the zucchini on a baking sheet and toss with olive oil. Sprinkle with Parmesan cheese, and salt and pepper. Roast until tender, about 15 minutes.

steak and zucchini shish kabobs

preparation time: 10 minutes

marinating time: 30 minutes

cook time: 10 minutes

total time: 50 minutes

1 (1-2 pound) sirloin steak

1 cup steak marinade

1 zucchini or yellow squash

½ cup cherry tomatoes

metal or soaked wooden skewers

Place the meat in a large plastic container or in a baking dish. Use a fork to poke holes all over the steak, and then cover with half the marinade. Flip over and cover with the remaining marinade. For maximum flavor, cover and refrigerate for 30 minutes or longer.

Meanwhile, heat the grill or grill pan to medium-high and cut the zucchini into 1-inch slices.

Cut the steak into cubes. Then thread the steak, zucchini, and tomatoes onto the skewers. Season with salt and pepper.

Clean and lightly oil the hot grill. Place the shish kabobs on the grill and cook for 10–15 minutes, or until the vegetables are tender and the steak is cooked to your liking. Flip occasionally as it cooks.

meat and other proteins

beans

Beans are extremely high in protein (about 14 grams per cup!), and generally low in fat and calories. Most beans are heart-healthy and rich in fiber, folates, and potassium. They are an excellent source of antioxidants, and may relieve constipation, combat fatigue, and reduce irritability. Some nutrition experts say they may reduce the risk of diabetes and cancer.

 Canned beans are easy and convenient. If you choose to use these, look for beans with low-sodium and a BPA-free liner.

bean baby food

START WITH 1 cup of dried beans or 1 (15-ounce) can of beans

1. prep

If using dried beans, pour them in a colander and sort through, throwing out any shriveled beans, stems, or small pebbles. Then rinse with water.

2. cook

If using canned beans, follow the cooking directions on the package. Then drain the water in a colander, and rinse the beans well. If using dried beans, choose from the following cooking methods.

BOIL

cook time: 1–2 hours

Place the dried beans in a saucepan and cover with 1–2 inches of water. Bring to a boil, and then reduce the heat to low and simmer. Cooking time will differ depending on the type of bean, but they usually take between 1–2 hours. Keep checking the pot during cooking to make sure the water level stays above the beans. Cook until the beans are tender and creamy. Then drain the excess water (or reserve some of the cooking liquid to thin the purees). Measure 1½ cups of prepared beans.

SLOW-COOK

cook time: 3 hours

Place the beans and 6 cups water in a slow cooker. Cook on high for 3–4 hours or on low for 6–8 hours. Keep an eye on the amount of water in the pot, making sure the water level stays above the beans. Cook until the beans are tender and creamy. Then drain the excess water (or reserve some of the cooking liquid to thin the purees). Measure 1½ cups of prepared beans.

3. add mix-ins & serve

Serve on its own or with tasty mix-ins. Puree, mash, or serve whole depending on your baby's stage.

simply bean puree

9 months +

MIX-INS

1½ tablespoons breast milk, formula, or water

Place beans and breast milk, formula, or water in a food processor and whirl to make a smooth puree with tiny lumps.

bean-butternut squash puree

10 months +

MIX-INS

1 cup winter squash, peeled and cubed

3 tablespoons breast milk, formula or water

Cook squash until tender (microwave for 5–10 minutes, boil or steam for 13 minutes, or roasted for 30 minutes at 400°F). Place the squash, beans, and breast milk, formula, or water in a food processor and pulse to make a chunky puree.

beans and avocado

11 months +

MIX-INS

½ avocado (about ¼ cup diced avocado)

Remove the avocado from the peel and finely dice. Mix the avocado and ¼ cup beans together in a small bowl and serve as finger food.

bean and corn salad

12 months +

MIX-INS

½ cup frozen sweet corn

Cook the corn as directed on the bag, until tender. Mix the corn and ½ cup of beans together in a small bowl and serve as finger food.

mama recipes

slow cooker pot of beans

total time: 3-8 hours

1 pound dried beans

3 quarts chicken stock

2 bay leaves

Place the beans in a colander and sort through, throwing out any shriveled beans, stems, or small pebbles. Then rinse with water.

Add the beans, stock, and bay leaves to a slow cooker. Cook on high for 3–4 hours or low for 6–8 hours until the beans are creamy. Keep an eye on the amount of stock in the pot, making sure the beans don't dry out. Freeze leftovers in individual portions for up to 6 months.

meat and other proteins

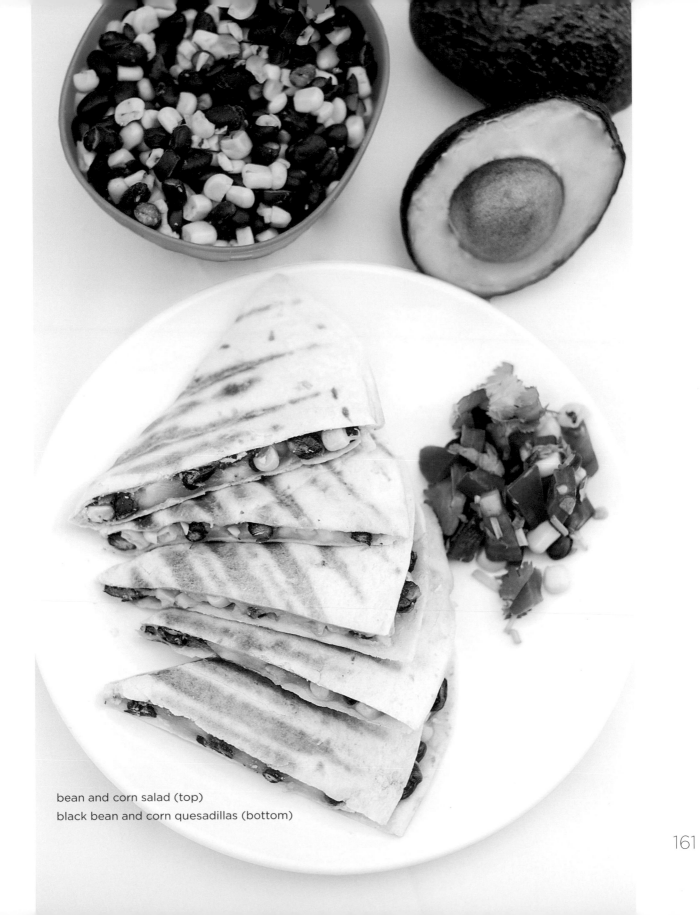

bean and corn salad (top)
black bean and corn quesadillas (bottom)

black bean and corn quesadillas

preparation time: 10 minutes

cook time: 10 minutes

¾ cup frozen corn

1 (15-ounce) can of black beans or 1 cup freshly cooked black beans

½ tablespoon butter

2 medium flour tortillas

1 cup Mexican cheese or cheddar cheese, shredded

¼ teaspoon taco seasoning

salsa, guacamole, or sour cream for dipping

Cook the corn as directed on the bag. Meanwhile, if using canned black beans, simmer in a saucepan until hot, about 5 minutes.

In a large skillet, heat half the butter over medium-high heat until melted. Then add the tortilla. Cook for 2 minutes to lightly brown and flip.

Place half of the black beans and corn onto one half of the tortilla, and then sprinkle with cheese and taco seasoning. Fold the other half of the tortilla over the stuffing and cook until golden brown on one side. Flip, and cook until the cheese has melted and the bottom is golden brown. Place on a serving plate. Use the remaining ingredients to make the second quesadilla.

Slice the quesadillas into quarters, and serve with dipping sauce.

tuscan chicken with cannelloni beans

preparation time: 5 minutes

cook time: 15 minutes

⅓ cup flour

2 thin chicken breasts

1 tablespoon olive oil

2 garlic cloves, diced

1 (15-ounce) can cannelloni beans, drained

1 medium tomato, chopped

2 tablespoons lemon juice

⅓ cup fresh basil, chopped

Place the flour in a bowl and coat both sides of the chicken in flour. Heat the oil in a skillet over medium heat and add the chicken and garlic. Cook for 3 minutes per side, or until the chicken has a light brown crust on both sides.

Add the beans and tomato to the skillet and simmer for 5 minutes, or until the chicken is cooked through and the beans are hot. If the skillet gets dry during cooking, add a tablespoon of water to keep it moist. Top with lemon juice and basil and season generously with salt and pepper.

Spoon the beans onto serving dishes and place the chicken on top.

curried chickpea salad sandwich

total time: 15 minutes

1 (15-ounce) can chickpeas or 1½ cups prepared chickpeas

⅓ cup carrots, peeled and diced

¼ cup raisins

¼ cup walnuts, chopped

¼ cup mayo

1½ teaspoon curry powder

1½ teaspoon lemon juice

4 slices bread or 2 pita

If using canned chickpeas, heat in a small saucepan until boiling. Then place in a colander and drain the water. Rinse with cold water to cool and pat the beans to remove as many of the shells as you can.

Meanwhile, dice the carrots and mix the raisins, walnuts, mayo, curry powder, and lemon juice together in a medium bowl.

Add the chickpeas to the bowl. Stir to combine. Roughly mash the chickpeas to a mix of mashed and semi-solid. Season with salt and pepper.

To serve, spoon the chickpea salad onto wheat bread or into a pita.

beef

Beef is an excellent source high-quality protein. Just one serving provides the entire recommended daily intake. It is also an excellent source of absorbable iron, zinc, and B vitamins. The nutrients in beef help with brain function, and red blood cell production. It provides energy, strengthens the immune system, and keeps you feeling full.

 If your budget allows, choose meat from grass-fed cows whenever possible. It may contain less fat, and a significantly more nutrients than conventional beef.

To prevent illness, cook beef well-done for baby.

beef baby food

START WITH ½ pound of ground beef or 1 (6-ounce) steak

1. prep
If using steak, trim away any excess fat.

2. cook
If using ground beef, heat a nonstick skillet over medium heat. Then add the meat. Break up the beef with a spatula and stir occasionally. Cook until the beef is browned and no longer pink, about 7–10 minutes. Drain excess grease. If using steak, choose from the following cooking methods.

SAUTÉ

cook time: 8 minutes.

Heat 2 teaspoons of oil in a sauté pan over medium-high heat. Place the steak in the pan, and cook for 4–6 minutes on each side. The steak should feel firm, and look gray-brown on the inside. Remove the steak from the pan and place on a cutting board. Let the steak rest for 5 minutes to allow the juices to settle. Cut into ½-inch cubes.

BAKE

cook time: 10 minutes

Preheat the oven to 375°F. Line a baking sheet with aluminum foil and spray with cooking spray.

Put the steak on the aluminum foil and place in the oven. Cook for 5 minutes per side, until well-done. Let the steak rest on a cutting board for 5 minutes before cutting it into ½-inch cubes.

BROIL

cook time: 10 minutes

Heat the broiler to medium-high. Line a baking sheet with aluminum foil and spray with cooking spray. Place the steak on the baking sheet and cook for 5–8 minutes per side, or until well-done. Let the steak rest on a cutting board for 5 minutes before cutting into ½-inch cubes.

GRILL

cook time: 12 minutes

Preheat grill to 350°F or the grill pan to medium. Lightly oil the grill grate with vegetable oil. Place the steak on the grate and cook for 6-8 minutes per side, until well-done. Let the steak rest on a cutting board for 5 minutes before cutting into ½-inch cubes.

3. add mix-ins and serve

Serve simply or with tasty mix-ins. Puree, shred, or finely dice according to your baby's stage.

simply beef puree

6 months +

MIX-INS

¼ cup + 2 tablespoons breast milk, formula, or water

Puree the beef and breast milk, formula, or water in a food processor until completely smooth and liquefied.

beef with green beans

7 months +

MIX-INS

¾ cup green beans, ends trimmed

¼ cup + 2 tablespoons breast milk, formula, or water

Cook the green beans until tender (microwave, boil, or steam for 3–7 minutes). Puree the beef and green beans and breast milk, formula, or water in a food processor until smooth.

beef, carrot, and parsnip puree

8 months +

MIX-INS

1 small carrot, peeled (about ½ cup)

1 small parsnip, peeled (about ½ cup)

¼ cup breast milk, formula, or water

Cut the carrot and parsnip into 2-inch pieces. Cook until tender (microwave for 3–6 minutes, steam or boil for 7–9 minutes, or roast for 25 minutes at 400°F). Place the cooked beef, carrots, and parsnips in a food processor to make a smooth, thick puree.

apricot glazed beef

9 months +

MIX-INS

¾ cup dried apricots

Place the apricots in a microwave-safe dish. Then cover with water and cook for 2 minutes, or until plump. Place the apricots, beef, and ¼ cup of cooking water in a food processor and puree to make a soft, lumpy puree.

creamy spinach and beef

10 months +

MIX-INS

2 cups fresh spinach, washed

3 tablespoons breast milk, formula, or water

Cook the spinach (microwave, sauté, boil, or steam for 2–4 minutes). Place the cooked beef, spinach, and breast milk, formula, or water in a food processor and puree to create a chunky puree.

first steak and potatoes

11 months +

MIX-INS

1 small potato

Cook the potato until tender (for the whole potato, microwave 9 minutes, chop and boil for 15 minutes, or roast for 30 minutes at 425°F). Cut the steak into small shreds, if using; or, break up ground beef into small bits. Dice the potato. Serve a few pieces of steak and potato a time as finger food.

baby beef taco

12 months +

MIX-INS

2 tablespoons shredded cheese

2 tablespoons tomato, finely chopped

Toss ½ cup of ground beef or finely diced steak in a bowl with the cheese and tomato. Serve as finger food.

mama recipes

skillet steaks with herb butter

preparation time: 5 minutes

cook time: 10 minutes

1 tablespoon butter

1 teaspoon Italian seasoning

2 boneless beef sirloin steaks

1 tablespoon olive oil

Place the butter in a microwave-safe dish and microwave for 8 seconds to soften. Use a fork to mash the herbs in the butter until fully combined. Then place back in the refrigerator.

Season the steak generously with salt and pepper. Heat the oil in a heavy skillet or Dutch oven over medium-high heat. Add the steak and cook for 4–5 minutes on each side, or until cooked to your liking.

Let the steak rest on a cutting board for 5 minutes. Then spread with herb butter and serve with veggies. (This dish is wonderful with creamed spinach.)

american beef tacos

preparation time: 5 minutes

cook time: 15 minutes

1 pound of ground beef

½ cup onion, chopped

1 pouch taco sauce

1 tomato

2 cups bagged romaine lettuce

1 cup shredded Mexican or cheddar cheese

taco shells

Heat a nonstick skillet over medium heat. Then add the ground beef and onion. Break up the beef with a spatula and stir occasionally. Cook until the beef is no longer pink, about 8 minutes. Stir in the sauce and cook for another minute.

Meanwhile, chop the tomato. Set up a taco buffet on your kitchen table, placing the lettuce, tomato, and cheese in their own bowls with a spoon. Warm the taco shells in the microwave or the oven as directed on the box. Then sit down and assemble the tacos as you like them.

perfectly grilled steak and potatoes

preparation time: 5 minutes

marinating time: 1 hour

cook time: 30 minutes

2 (6-ounce) beef steaks

½ cup steak marinade

2 russet potatoes

1 tablespoon olive oil

½ tablespoon Italian seasoning

Place the meat in a large plastic container or baking dish. Use a fork to poke holes all over the steak. Then cover with half the marinade. Flip over and cover with the remaining marinade. For maximum flavor, cover and refrigerate for one hour or longer.

Meanwhile, chop the potatoes into 1-inch cubes and place them in a bowl. Toss with olive oil and Italian seasoning until completely coated. Season generously with salt and pepper. Place the potatoes in the center of a sheet of foil. Fold to make a closed square packet, then seal the edges.

Preheat the grill to 350°F. When the steaks have only 15 minutes left to marinate, place the potato foil packet on the grill to start cooking. Cook the potatoes for 30 minutes, or until fork tender, flipping halfway through.

When the steak is finished marinating, oil the grill grates, and place the steak on the grill for 3–5 minutes per side, or until cooked to your liking. Let the steak rest on a cutting board or plate for 5 minutes before serving to keep the juices inside. Take the packets off the grill, and scoop the potatoes onto serving plates with the steak.

chicken

Skinless chicken is an excellent source of high-quality, lean protein and B vitamins. It helps boost energy, keeps your heart, nervous system, and digestive tract healthy, and stabilizes mood. The nutrients in chicken promote healthy hair, skin, and joints, and reduce symptoms of PMS. Though dark meat has a higher fat content, it also contains more minerals.

 Always check that chicken is cooked through before serving (by cutting into it with a knife). The meat should look opaque and white, not pink. The juices should also run clear. If you're unsure if chicken is done, use a meat thermometer to check the internal temperature. Thoroughly cooked chicken should read 165°F or above.

Choose natural, unprocessed chicken whenever you can. You can tell that chicken is processed if there are additives listed on the label, such as MSG or sodium erythorbate.

chicken baby food

START WITH one (6-ounce) skinless chicken breast or 2 chicken tenderloins

1. prep

Trim the fat, connective tissue, and cartilage from chicken breast.

2. cook

Choose from the following cooking methods.

SAUTÉ

cook time: 10 minutes

Heat 2 teaspoons of oil in a sauté pan over medium-high heat. Then add the chicken and cook for 5 minutes per side, or until the chicken is opaque throughout.

GRILL

cook time: 12 minutes

Preheat the grill to 350°F. Lightly oil the grill grate with vegetable oil and place the chicken on the grill. Grill for 6–8 minutes per side, or until the chicken is opaque throughout.

POACH

cook time: 10 minutes

Bring 2 cups of water to a boil in a medium saucepan. Add the chicken, then cover and cook for 10 minutes, or until opaque throughout.

meat and other proteins

BAKE

cook time: 10 minutes

Preheat the oven to 375°F. Spray a baking dish lightly with cooking spray. Then add the chicken. Bake for 10–15 minutes, or until cooked through.

3. add mix-ins & serve

Serve on its own or with tasty mix-ins. Puree, shred, or finely dice according to your baby's stage.

simply chicken puree

6 months +

MIX-INS

¼ cup + 2 tablespoons breast milk, formula, or water

Puree the cooked chicken and breast milk, formula, or water in a blender until smooth and soupy.

chicken with apples

7 months +

MIX-INS

1 large apple, peeled and halved

¼ cup + 2 tablespoons breast milk, formula, or water

Cook the apple until tender (microwave for 3 minutes, boil for 10 minutes, steam for 12 minutes, or bake for 15 minutes at 375°F). Place the apple and chicken, and breast milk, formula, or water in a blender and whirl until smooth.

chicken, carrots, and brown rice

8 months +

MIX-INS

7 baby carrots

⅓ cup cooked brown rice

¼ cup breast milk, formula, or water

Cook the carrots until tender (microwave for 3–6 minutes, steam or boil for 7 minutes, or roast for 25 minutes at 400°F). Place the chicken, carrots, brown rice, and breast milk, formula, or water in a blender. Whirl to create a smooth and thick puree.

chicken-sweet potato puree

9 months +

MIX-INS

1 small sweet potato

⅓ cup breast milk, formula, or water

Pierce the potato all over with a fork. Then cook the potato until tender (microwave for 9 minutes or bake for 1 hour at 350°F). When the potato is cool to touch, cut it in half, then scoop out the potato flesh. Place the chicken and sweet potato, and breast milk, formula, or water in a blender and puree until mashed with tiny lumps.

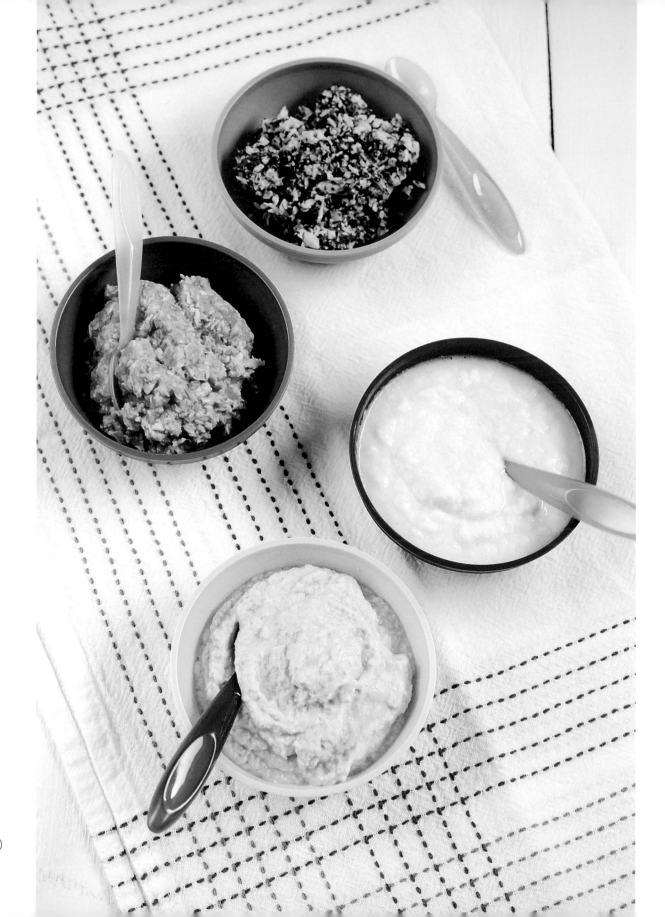

chicken-sweet pea mash

10 months +

MIX-INS

½ cup frozen sweet peas, thawed

¾ cup breast milk, formula, or water

Cook the peas until tender (microwave for 2 minutes or steam or boil for 3 minutes). Pulse the cooked chicken and peas, and breast milk, formula, or water in a blender to create a chunky puree.

chicken, blueberry, and spinach puree

11 months +

MIX-INS

½ cup blueberries

4 cups fresh spinach

Wash blueberries and spinach thoroughly. Cook the spinach (microwave for 2 minutes, steam for 4–6 minutes on the stovetop, or boil for 5 minutes). Place the chicken, blueberries, and spinach in a blender and whirl to create a chunky puree.

chicken strips

12 months +

Cut the cooked chicken into thin strips, about the size of your pinky finger. Serve 1 or 2 pieces at a time. Keep an eye on baby, making sure he doesn't shove the whole thing in his mouth or take too big of a bite.

(facing page, clockwise from top)
chicken, blueberry, and spinach puree;
simply chicken puree, chicken with apples;
and chicken-sweet potato puree

coconut chicken tenders

preparation time: 15 minutes

cook time: 15 minutes

This is one of my family's go-to recipes. We make it when family is in town, and everyone always cleans their plates. Serve with fresh steamed broccoli for a complete meal.

1 lb. chicken tenders

½ cup flour

1 teaspoon cayenne

¾ cup panko bread crumbs

¾ cup sweetened, shredded coconut

2 eggs, beaten

1 tablespoon milk

sweet chili sauce for dipping

Preheat the oven to 425°F, and line a baking sheet with aluminum foil. Spritz with cooking spray.

Set up your breading station. Stir together the flour and cayenne in one bowl, the panko and coconut in another bowl, and the egg and milk each in separate bowls.

Dunk the chicken in the flour and shake off the excess. Next dunk the chicken in the egg, and then in the coconut mixture to coat. Repeat with the remaining chicken strips.

Arrange the chicken tenders on the baking sheet in a single layer. Cook for 12 minutes, until cooked through. Then flip the tenders and broil on high for about 3 minutes or until crispy. Serve with steamed broccoli and sweet chili dipping sauce.

roasted chicken with vegetables

preparation time: 10 minutes

cook time: 60 minutes

This one-pan dinner can be made in its entirety before company comes over. When your guests arrive and want time with the baby, you can enjoy a much-needed mommy break!

When you're at the grocery store, look for a ready to cook roasting chicken, or ask your butcher to prepare the chicken for cooking (remove the giblets and rinse out the inside). That way it saves you those steps at home.

1 cup baby carrots

2 potatoes, chopped

4 tablespoons olive oil

1 pack of fresh poultry herbs

1 (2 –3 pound) roasting chicken

½ lemon

½ onion, peeled

1 slice bread

Preheat the oven to 425°F. Toss the carrots, potatoes, and 2 tablespoons of olive oil in the bottom of a roasting pan. Place a sprig of fresh herbs on top.

Place the chicken on a cutting board and pat dry with a paper towel. Brush the bird with olive oil (about 2 tablespoons), and season generously with salt and pepper. Cut the lemon and onion halves so that they fit into the chicken. Then place the onion, lemon, and herbs inside the chicken. Squish a piece of bread over the hole to cover it.

Place the roasting rack over the vegetables. Add the chicken to the rack and tuck the wings underneath.

Cook for 1 hour, or until the temperature reaches 165°F and the juices run clear. Take the chicken out of the oven and cover with foil. Let it sit for 15 minutes before carving. Remove the herbs from the vegetables before serving.

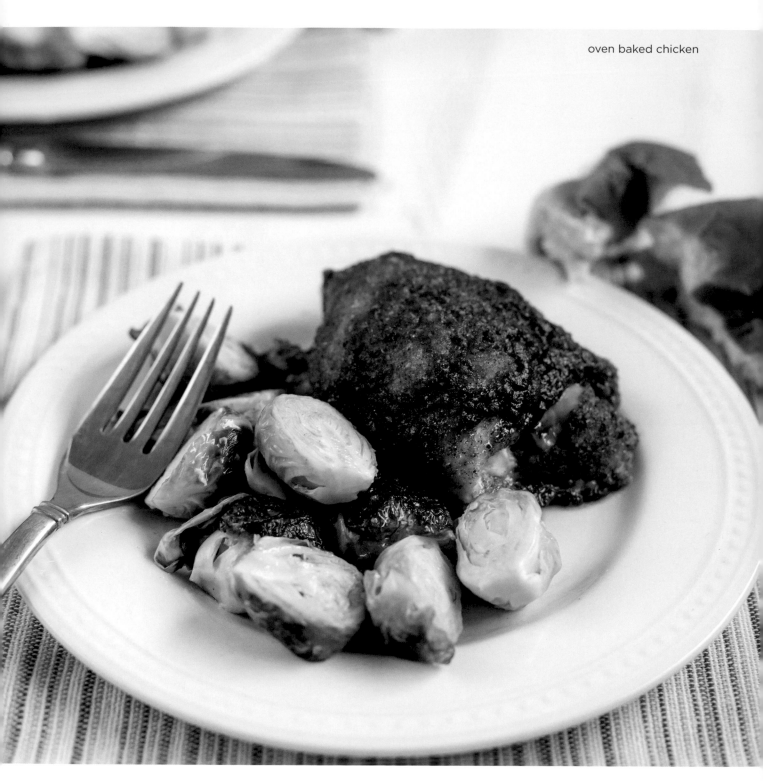

meat and other proteins

oven baked chicken

preparation time: 5 minutes

cook time: 30 minutes

2 large chicken thighs

1–1½ teaspoons Jamaican jerk seasoning

1 tablespoon brown sugar

Preheat the oven to 400°F. Line a baking sheet with aluminum foil and spray with nonstick cooking spray. Place the chicken on the baking sheet skin-side up.

Dry the top of the chicken with a paper towel. Then coat it generously with jerk seasoning. Press the brown sugar onto the skin, and then season with salt and pepper.

Bake for 25–35 minutes, or until the skin is crispy. A meat thermometer should read 165°F by the bone. Serve with a side of vegetables.

cranberry chicken salad

preparation time: 10 minutes

Store-bought rotisserie chicken makes this a super easy salad, but you can also cook up an extra chicken breast at dinner instead. Make the salad the night before for a fast and easy lunch.

1 cup cooked chicken breast, chopped

¼ cup dried cranberries

½ cup sliced celery, sliced

½ cup diced apple, finely diced

¼ cup mayonnaise

4 slices bread, 2 croissants, or 2 lettuce cups

In a medium bowl, mix together the chicken, cranberries, celery, apple, and mayonnaise. Season with salt and pepper.

Spoon the chicken salad onto a slice of bread or croissant and top it with the remaining piece. Alternatively, wrap in the lettuce cup.

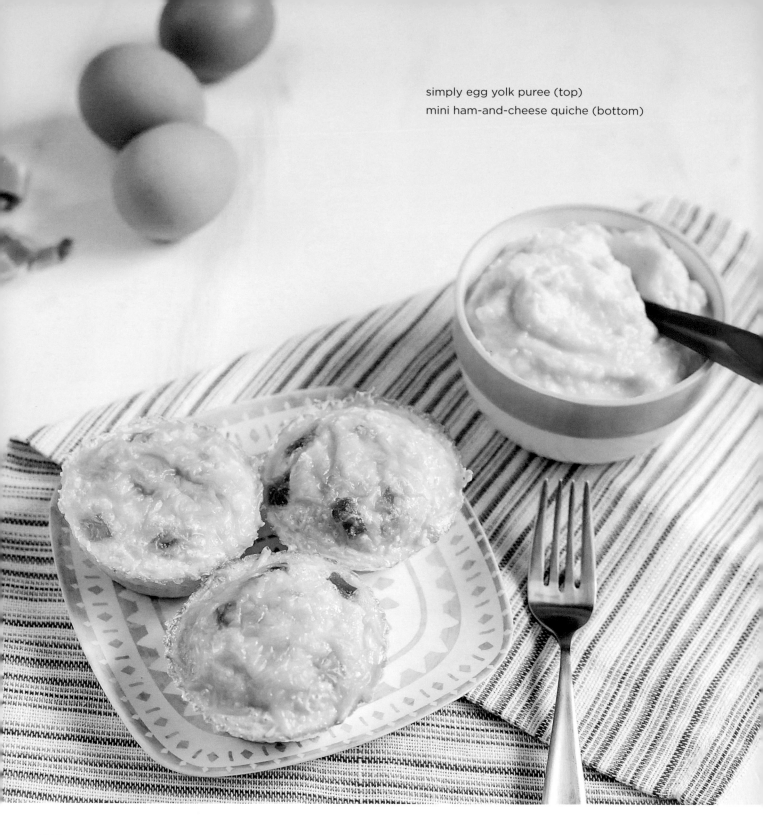

simply egg yolk puree (top)
mini ham-and-cheese quiche (bottom)

meat and other proteins

eggs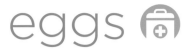

Eggs are an excellent source of protein, vitamins A and B, potassium, and selenium. These nutrients help keep the eyes, heart, brain, and cell membranes healthy. Eggs also keep you feeling satiated (making them a great breakfast), boost energy and mood, and may help prevent breast cancer and cardiovascular disease.

 Choose organic, free-range eggs whenever possible. They tend to be more nutritious and are less likely to be contaminated by salmonella.

egg yolk baby food

START WITH 4 large whole eggs

1. cook

Choose from the following cooking methods.

BOIL

cook time: 12 minutes

Place the eggs in a medium saucepan, and cover with an inch of water. Bring to a full boil. Then turn off the heat and cover. Let sit for 12 minutes. Using a slotted spoon, remove the eggs and place in a large bowl. Add cold water and ice. Allow the eggs to cool for 10 minutes. Remove the shell and egg white and set aside or discard.

STEAM

cook time: 22 minutes

Set up a steamer basket in a medium pot and add water so it reaches just below the basket. Bring to a boil. Add the eggs, then cover and steam for 22 minutes. Using a slotted spoon, remove the eggs and place in a large bowl. Add cold water and ice. Allow the eggs cool for 10 minutes. Remove the shell and egg white, and set aside or discard.

2. add mix-ins & serve

Serve simply or with tasty mix-ins. Puree, mash, or dice according to your baby's stage.

simply egg yolk puree
8 months +

MIX-INS

2 tablespoons breast milk, formula, or water

In a small bowl, mash the egg yolk with breast milk, formula, or water to form a smooth, thick puree.

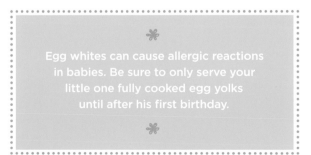

Egg whites can cause allergic reactions in babies. Be sure to only serve your little one fully cooked egg yolks until after his first birthday.

steak and egg yolk

9 months +

MIX-INS

3 beef-steak cubes

Cook the steak well done (sauté for 8 minutes, broil for 10 minutes, or bake for 10 minutes at 375°F). Finely shred the steak and dice the egg or place in a food processor and blitz.

egg yolk and rice

10 months +

MIX-INS

3 tablespoons cooked brown rice

1 tablespoon breast milk, formula, or water

In a small bowl, mix the egg yolk and rice, and breast milk, formula, or water together until combined.

egg yolk and potatoes

11 months +

MIX-INS

¼ cup frozen diced white potato

Cook the potatoes as directed on the package. Finely chop the egg yolk and potatoes. Serve as finger food.

baby's first ham and egg yolk

12 months +

MIX-INS

1 slice deli ham

Heat the ham in a skillet with a dab of butter until caramelized. Dice the ham and egg yolk, and mix together in a small bowl and serve as finger food.

mama recipes

mini ham-and-cheese quiche

preparation time: 10 minutes

cook time: 25 minutes

Cook once and eat twice with this tasty and satisfying egg breakfast.

8 eggs

2 slices deli ham, diced

½ cup cheddar cheese

Preheat the oven to 375°F. Spray a muffin pan with cooking spray, or put 8 silicone cupcake liners into a muffin pan and spray with cooking spray.

Whisk the eggs in a medium bowl until combined, and pour into a liquid measuring cup (to make it easier to pour). Scoop about a tablespoon each of ham and cheese into the bottom of 8 muffin tins. Top the ham and cheese with the egg mixture, pouring equally among the tins.

Bake for 25 minutes, or until the eggs have risen and are puffy and golden on top. Store leftovers in the refrigerator. Heat in the microwave for a fast breakfast the next day.

scrambled omelet on toast

total time: 10 minutes

Omelets are extremely versatile. Use whatever you have in your kitchen as a filling—cheese, herbs, veggies, or meat.

4 eggs

½ tablespoon butter

⅓ cup filling (cheese, spinach, sautéed mushrooms, etc.)

4 slices bread, toasted

Crack the eggs into a medium bowl. Then beat together until combined.

In a nonstick skillet, heat the butter over medium heat until melted. If using an ingredient in the filling that needs to be cooked, add it to the skillet and cook through. Then pour the egg mixture into the pan along with any additional toppings. Cook, stirring often, until the eggs are set. Place over toast.

classic egg salad sandwich

preparation time: 5 minutes

4 hard-boiled eggs, peeled

¼ cup mayonnaise

1 teaspoon white vinegar

1 teaspoon prepared yellow mustard

sprinkle of paprika

4 slices whole wheat bread

In a medium bowl, finely chop the eggs with a knife. Stir in the mayonnaise, vinegar, mustard, and paprika. Season with salt and pepper.

Spoon the egg mixture onto two pieces of bread, and top with the remaining slices to make sandwiches.

southwestern breakfast skillet

preparation time: 5 minutes
cook time: 15 minutes

If you use frozen potatoes and peppers it whips up in a flash. It's a well-deserved, weekend treat!

2 tablespoons canola oil

3 cups frozen diced potatoes

1 cup frozen sliced bell peppers

1 teaspoon creole seasoning

6 eggs

½ cup shredded cheddar cheese

Preheat the oven to 375°F. Drop the sealed bag of potatoes on the floor a couple of times to loosen them if they are frozen in a clump.

Heat the oil in a Dutch oven or oven-proof skillet over medium-high heat on the stove. Add the potatoes and bell peppers. Sprinkle with creole seasoning, salt, and pepper. Cook until the potatoes are golden and tender, about 10 minutes.

Crack the eggs over the hash. Check to make sure there are no shell pieces in the dish. Top with cheese.

Cover and move to the oven. Bake until the egg whites are set and the yolk is to your liking, about 5–10 minutes.

fish

Fish is an excellent source of vitamins, antioxidants, and protein. It's particularly nutritious for nursing women and children. The Omega-3 fatty acids in fish may help ease symptoms of postpartum depression by boosting mood, memory, and concentration. It may also reduce risk of all sorts of health issues, like heart disease, cancer, diabetes, Alzheimer's, and more. The USDA recommends that nursing women eat seafood twice a week.[34]

The nutrients in fish are wonderful for infants as well. They promote healthy growth and brain development, and may reduce the risk of autism, attention deficit and hyperactivity disorder, and dyslexia.

To save yourself some time, ask the fishmonger at the grocery store to remove the pin bones and skin from fish fillets. If a fishmonger isn't available, you can do it at home by running your hand along the fillet and pulling the bones out, and using a knife to slice off the skin.

Like all meats, fish should be cooked well-done for baby. To tell if fish is cooked properly, insert a fork into the thickest part, and pull it back so you can see the meat. Undercooked fish will be jelly-like and see-through, while properly cooked fish will be opaque and flake apart with the fork. If you still aren't sure if the fish is done, use a meat thermometer and check that the thickest part reads 145°F or above.

fish baby food

START WITH 1 (6-ounce) fresh or frozen fish fillet

1. prep

Remove all the bones and skin if they haven't been removed already.

2. cook

If using frozen fish, follow the directions on the package. If using fresh fish, choose one of the cooking methods that follow.

MICROWAVE

cook time: 4 minutes

Spray a microwave-safe dish with cooking spray. Add the fish, then cover, leaving an air vent for the steam. Cook for 4 minutes on high, and then check to see if it's done. If it needs more time, continue cooking for 30-second intervals until fully cooked, then chop.

POACH

cook time: 5 minutes

Fill half of a medium saucepan with water and bring to a boil. Add the fish, then cover and simmer for 5–10 minutes, or until cooked through. Roughly chop.

SAUTÉ

cook time: 5 minutes

Heat a sauté pan over medium heat, then add a tablespoon of butter or oil. Add the fish and cook for 5 minutes, flipping halfway through until the fish is fully cooked. Then chop.

GRILL OR GRILL PAN

cook time: 10 minutes

Preheat the grill to 350°F or a grill pan to medium Oil the grates, then add the fish to the grill and cover and cook for 5 minutes per side, or until fish is fully cooked. Then chop.

BAKE

cook time: 10 minutes

Preheat the oven to 400°F. Spray a baking dish with cooking spray, then add the fish. Bake for 10–15 minutes, until the fish is fully cooked, then chop.

3. add mix-ins & serve

Serve on its own or with tasty mix-ins. Puree, flake, or dice according to your baby's stage.

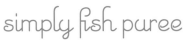

simply fish puree

6 months +

MIX-INS

¼ cup breast milk, formula, or water

Puree the fish and breast milk, formula, or water in a blender until smooth and liquefied.

fish-peach puree

7 months +

MIX-INS

1 peach

¼ cup breast milk, formula or water

Cook the peach until tender (microwave for 2 minutes, steam for 5 minutes, or boil for 8–10 minutes). When cool to the touch, peel the skin off the peach and chop. Puree the peach and fish, and breast milk, formula, or water in a food processor until smooth.

> ✳
>
> Shop smart and only choose fish that's low in mercury and contaminants. Hold off on feeding baby any type of shellfish until after his first birthday.
>
> low mercury fish (eat these):
> salmon, tilapia, shrimp, trout, catfish, flounder, haddock, perch, sole
>
> high mercury fish (don't eat these):
> king mackerel, marlin, shark, tilefish, swordfish, bigeye or ahi tuna
>
> ✳

fish chowder

8 months +

MIX-INS

½ cup frozen peas and carrots

3 tablespoons breast milk, formula, or water

Cook the peas and carrots as directed on the bag. Combine the peas, carrots, fish, and breast milk, formula, or water in a food processor and whirl to form a smooth puree.

fish and zucchini puree

9 months +

MIX-INS

¾ cup zucchini, peeled and sliced

3 tablspoons breast milk, formula, or water

Cook the zucchini until tender (microwave for 5 minutes, grill in a foil packet, steam, or sauté for 8 minutes, or roast for 15 minutes at 450°F). Place the fish, zucchini, and breast milk, formula, or water in a food processor and whirl create a soft, lumpy puree.

fish with creamy sauce

10 months +

MIX-INS

⅛ cup softened full-fat cream cheese

1 tablespoon breast milk, formula, or water

Leave the cream cheese out until it softens, or soften in the microwave. Place the fish and cream cheese, and breast milk, formula, or water in a blender and pulse until combined, forming a chunky puree.

fish with asparagus

11 months +

MIX-INS

5 asparagus, trimmed

Cook the asparagus until tender (microwave for 2 minutes, boil for 3 minutes, steam for 4 minutes, or roast for 15 minutes at 400°F). Pulse the fish and asparagus in a food processor until finely diced.

fish with broccoli and wild rice

12 months +

MIX-INS

¼ cup cooked broccoli

¼ cup cooked wild rice

This recipe is meant to be paired with the adult recipe that follows. Finely dice the broccoli and fish into bite-sized pieces. In a small bowl, stir the broccoli, rice, and ⅓ cup of fish together. Serve as finger food.

teriyaki salmon

preparation time: 5 minutes

cook time: 15 minutes

2 (6-ounce) salmon fillets, skinned and deboned

½ cup bottled teriyaki sauce

Preheat the oven to 400°F, and spray a baking dish with cooking spray. Place the fillets on the dish and cover with teriyaki sauce.

Bake for 15–25 minutes, or until the fish is flaky and opaque inside.

fish with broccoli and wild rice (top)
teriyaki salmon (bottom)

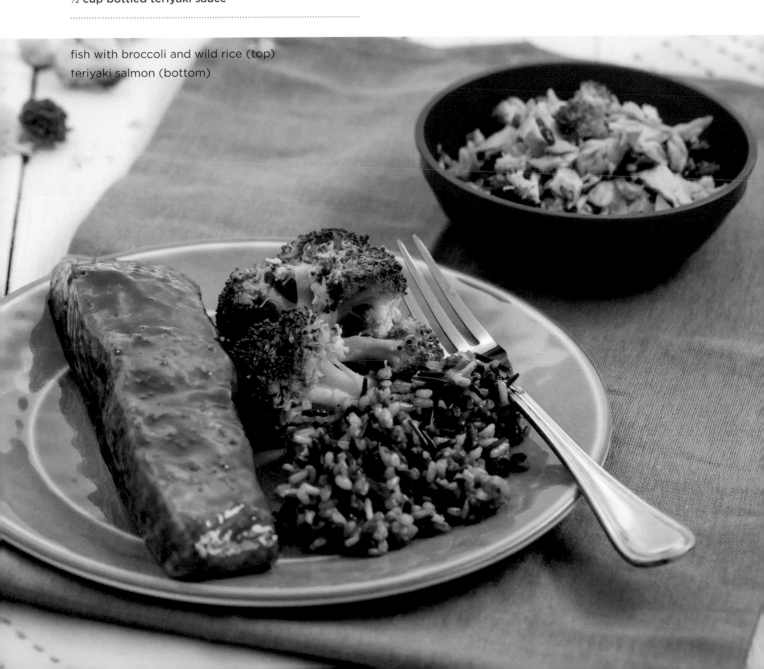

salmon wrapped in puff pastry

preparation time: 15 minutes

cook time: 25 minutes

Impress a loved one for a special occasion (or on a whim!) with this fancy looking dish. It's simple to put together and tastes amazing. If you need to, you can even prepare it earlier in the day and store it in the refrigerator until you're ready for dinner.

4 frozen puff pastry squares, thawed

4 tablespoons cream cheese, diced

2 (6-ounce) skinned and deboned salmon fillets, cubed

2 tablespoons coarsely chopped tarragon

1 egg

Preheat the oven to 400°F and line a baking sheet with parchment paper.

Roll the puff pastry out with a rolling pin so each is ⅛-inch thick. Mix the salmon and tarragon together, then place ½ of the salmon mixture in the center of each puff square. Top each with ½ the cream cheese, then top with the remaining pastry squares. Wrap the pastry around the salmon, making a package. Seal tightly.

Make an egg wash to create a shiny glow. Beat the egg with one tablespoon of cold water. Then brush the mixture over the top of each pie. Slice a few small slits into the top of the pies.

Use a large spatula to carefully transfer the pies, sealed-side down, onto the prepared baking sheet. Bake for 25 minutes, or until golden brown.

blackened tilapia with wild rice pilaf

preparation time: 5 minutes

cook time: 30 minutes

1 (6.3 ounce) box long-grain and wild rice

2 tilapia fillets, skinned and deboned

blackened fish seasoning

2 tablespoons unsalted butter

Begin cooking the wild rice as directed on the package. Meanwhile, coat both sides of the fillets with blackened fish seasoning.

When the rice has 10 minutes left, heat the butter in a nonstick skillet over medium-high heat. Add the fish and cook for 2–3 minutes per side, or until flaky and opaque inside. Serve the fish with a side of rice.

pork

Pork is high in protein, B vitamins, iron, and zinc. These nutrients help clear the skin, boost energy and metabolism, support healthy liver and lungs, and balance cholesterol.

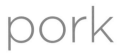 It can be tricky to tell when pork is done because it sometimes looks pink inside when it's fully cooked. The best way to tell if pork is properly cooked is to use a meat thermometer. Cook pork chops to 145°F for you and 160°F for baby.

pork baby food

START WITH 2 thin-cut, boneless pork chops

1. prep

Trim the excess fat from the pork chops.

2. cook

Choose from the following cooking methods.

SAUTÉ

cook time: 8 minutes

Heat 2 teaspoons of oil in a sauté pan, and add the pork chops. Sauté the pork for approximately 4 minutes per side, or until golden brown and cooked through. Let the pork rest to keep the juices inside, then chop.

BROIL

cook time: 10 minutes

Heat the broiler to medium-high, and then line a baking sheet with aluminum foil. Spray with cooking spray. Place the pork chops on the baking sheet and broil for 5 minutes per side, or until fully cooked. Let the pork rest to keep the juices inside, then chop.

BAKE

cook time: 15 minutes

Preheat the oven to 350°F. Line a baking sheet with aluminum foil, and then spray with cooking spray. Place the pork chop on the baking sheet and bake for 15 minutes, or until fully cooked. Flip halfway through. Let the pork rest to keep the juices inside, then chop.

3. add mix-ins & serve

Serve simply or with tasty mix-ins. Puree, shred, or finely dice according to your baby's stage.

simply pork puree

9 months +

MIX-INS

¼ cup + 2 tablespoons breast milk, formula, or water

Puree the pork and breast milk, formula, or water in a blender to create a soft, lumpy puree.

pork with peaches

10 months +

MIX-INS

1 peach

2 tablespoons breast milk, formula, or water

Cut the peach in half and remove the pit. Cook the peach until tender (microwave for 2 minutes, steam for 5 minutes, or boil for 8–10 minutes). When the peach is cool, peel off the skin. Place the pork and peach, and breast milk, formula, or water in a food processor and whirl to create a chunky puree.

sweet potato, apple, and pork

11 months +

MIX-INS

1 sweet potato

1 small apple

3 tablespoons breast milk, formula, or water

Peel and chop the sweet potato and apple. Start cooking the sweet potatoes, either in the microwave (cook for 9 minutes) or oven (roast for 30 minutes at 425°F). Toss the apples with the sweet potatoes and continue cooking both until tender, about 2 minutes in the microwave or 10 in the oven. Puree the pork, sweet potato, and apple in a food processor to create a chunky puree.

pork, snow peas, and brown rice

12 months +

MIX-INS

¼ cup frozen snow peas, thawed

2 tablespoons cooked brown rice

This recipe is meant to be paired with the adult recipe that follows. Cook the snow peas until tender (microwave for 3 minutes, or sauté or steam for 5 minutes). Meanwhile, finely dice one portion of the the pork into bite-sized pieces, and pop the peas out of the shell, if desired. Stir the pork, snow peas, and brown rice together in a bowl.

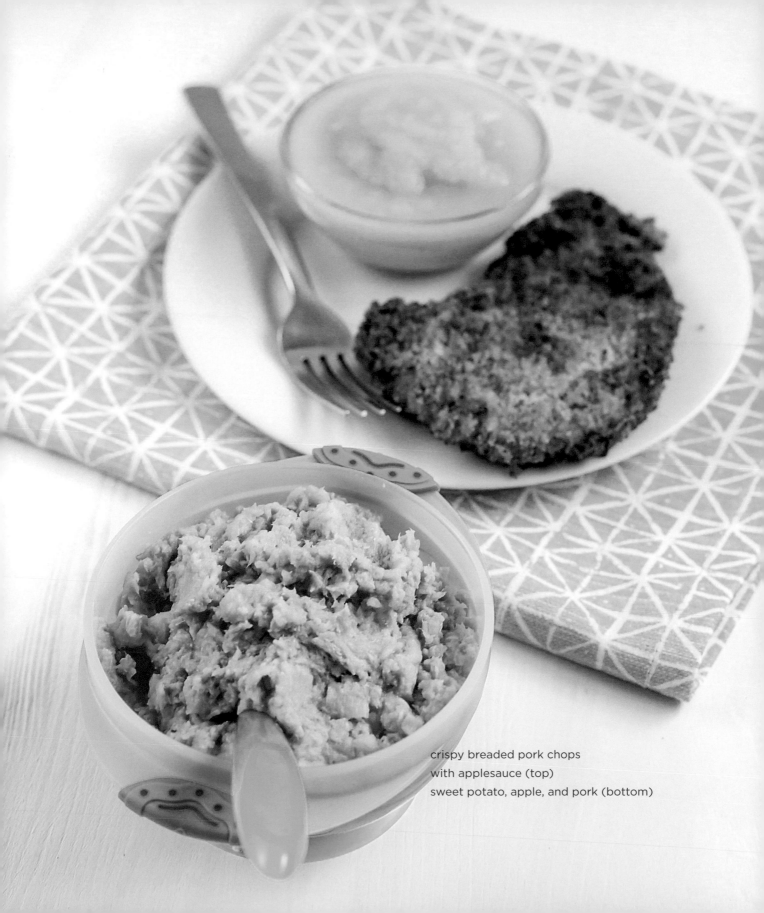

crispy breaded pork chops
with applesauce (top)
sweet potato, apple, and pork (bottom)

crispy breaded pork chops with applesauce

preparation time: 10 minutes

cook time: 10 minutes

4 thin-cut pork chops

¾ cup flour

1 cup panko bread crumbs

1 egg, beaten

½ teaspoon dried thyme

3 tablespoons canola oil

1 cup applesauce for serving

Season the pork with salt and pepper. Then put the flour, panko, and egg in separate bowls. Add the thyme to the flour and stir to combine.

Coat both sides of the pork chops in flour, then egg, then panko. Firmly press the panko onto the pork so it's well coated.

Heat the oil over medium heat in a nonstick skillet. When the oil is hot, add the pork chops and cook until golden brown and crispy, 4–5 minutes per side. Serve with veggies (this one is great with sweet potatoes or winter squash!) and applesauce.

sweet chili pork stir-fry

preparation time: 5 minutes

cook time: 25 minutes

1 cup brown or jasmine rice

2 cups frozen snow peas

1 garlic clove

3 tablespoons fresh basil leaves

3 teaspoons canola oil

2 pork chops

3 tablespoons sweet chili sauce

Cook the rice as directed on the bag. Meanwhile, thaw the snow peas, mince the garlic, and thinly slice the basil.

With 15 minutes left on the rice, heat the oil in a nonstick skillet over high heat. Add the pork chops, and cook, flipping halfway through, about 6 minutes. Remove from the pan and cut into thin strips.

Toss the garlic and snow peas into the skillet and stir-fry until tender-crisp, about 3 minutes. Then add the sliced pork and sweet chili sauce. Simmer until the sauce is hot and bubbling. Then stir in the basil. Serve over rice.

tofu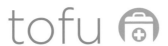

Tofu is an excellent source of plant-based protein, offering about 10 grams of protein in every ½ cup! It contains all eight essential amino acids, and is rich in both calcium and manganese. Tofu promotes strong bones and teeth, helps reduce symptoms of PMS, and lowers bad LDL cholesterol. It may even reduce the risk of cancer and heart disease.

Tofu is a man-made product derived from soy beans. Soy milk is curdled and pressed into a solid block in a process similar to how other kinds of milk are made into cheese. Tofu is usually refrigerated, and comes in different consistencies. Silken tofu is soft and creamy, making it great for purees and puddings. Firm and extra firm tofu works well as finger food for baby. It's also best for grilling, baking, and stir-frying. Tofu does not need to be cooked, but doing so gives it more flavor and texture.

tofu baby food

START WITH 1 cup silken or firm tofu

1. prep

Drain the excess water from the package. If using firm tofu, cut it into ⅓-inch slabs and pat them dry with a paper towel (7 strips = 1 cup).

2. cook

Tofu doesn't need to be cooked, and doesn't work well with silken tofu, but it can add flavor and texture to firm tofu. If using firm tofu, choose a cooking method from the following.

GRILL

cook time: 4 minutes

Heat the grill to medium, then rub the grill grates with vegetable oil. Place the tofu sticks on the grill and cook 2–3 minutes per side until crispy.

BROIL

cook time: 10 minutes

Preheat the broiler to high. Spray a rimmed baking sheet or baking dish with cooking spray. Add the tofu. Broil, flipping once, about 10 minutes or until the edges are golden brown.

SAUTÉ

cook time: 10 minutes

In a nonstick skillet, heat oil over medium-high heat. Add the tofu and pan fry until golden brown and crispy, about 5 minutes. Then flip and cook the other side to form a crust.

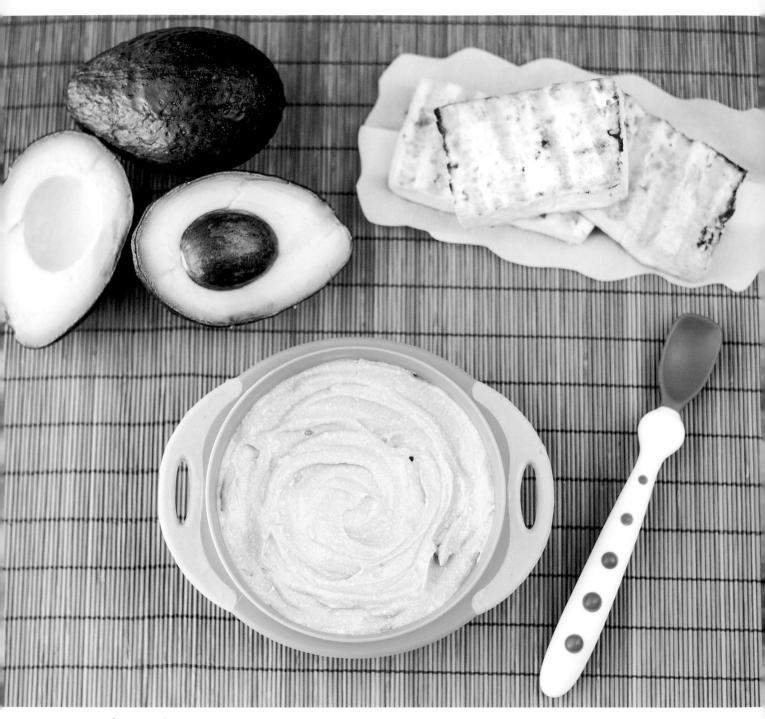

tofu-avocado puree

meat and other proteins

3. add mix-ins & serve

tofu-avocado puree

8 months +

MIX-INS

1 avocado

3 tablespoons breast milk, formula, or water

Cut the avocado in half from top to bottom, twisting both sides so it comes apart. Then scoop out the inside, discarding the seed. Puree the avocado and tofu, and breast milk, formula, or water in a food processor to create a thick and smooth puree.

banana-tofu puree

9 months +

MIX-INS

1 banana, peeled

2 tablespoons breast milk, formula, or water

Puree the tofu and banana, and breast milk, formula, or water in a food processor to create a soft puree with tiny lumps.

mango tofu with wheat germ

10 months +

MIX-INS

1 cup chopped mango

½ tablespoon wheat germ

Place the mango, tofu, and wheat germ in a food processor and pulse to create a chunky puree.

blueberry tofu

11 months +

MIX-INS

1 cup blueberries

Wash the blueberries thoroughly. Puree the blueberries and tofu in a food processor until smooth, or finely dice the blueberries and firm tofu, mix together, and serve as finger food. For a single serving, just mix an equal portion of diced tofu with blueberries.

tofu and zucchini

12 months +

MIX-INS

¼ cup zucchini

Sauté the zucchini until tender. Finely dice the zucchini and ¼ cup firm tofu (if using), and then stir together in a small bowl. Serve as finger food. Roughly puree if using silken tofu.

peanut noodles with tofu

preparation time: 5 minutes

cook time: 30 minutes

½ box soba (buckwheat) noodles or whole grain linguine

¾ cup teriyaki sauce

2 tablespoons peanut butter

3 tablespoons canola oil

1 (14-ounce) package of tofu, cut into 1-inch cubes

1 (12-ounce) package frozen Asian vegetables

¼ cup peanuts, as a garnish

Start cooking the noodles as directed on the box. Meanwhile, in a small bowl whisk the teriyaki sauce and peanut butter together until combined.

In a medium nonstick skillet, heat 2 tablespoons of oil over medium-high heat. Add the tofu. Pan fry until golden brown and crispy on one side, about 6–8 minutes. Resist your urge to flip the tofu before it is completely golden brown; it helps the crust develop if you let it be.

Flip, then cook the opposite side of the tofu until it forms a golden crust. Place the tofu in a bowl and cover to keep warm.

Add the remaining oil and frozen vegetables to the hot skillet. Cook until tender crisp, about 5 minutes. Pour the peanut sauce into the pan and stir to coat the vegetables. Cook until the sauce is hot and bubbling. If the sauce is too thin, whisk in 1 or 2 teaspoons of cornstarch. Turn off the burner and stir in the noodles. Serve and top with tofu and peanuts.

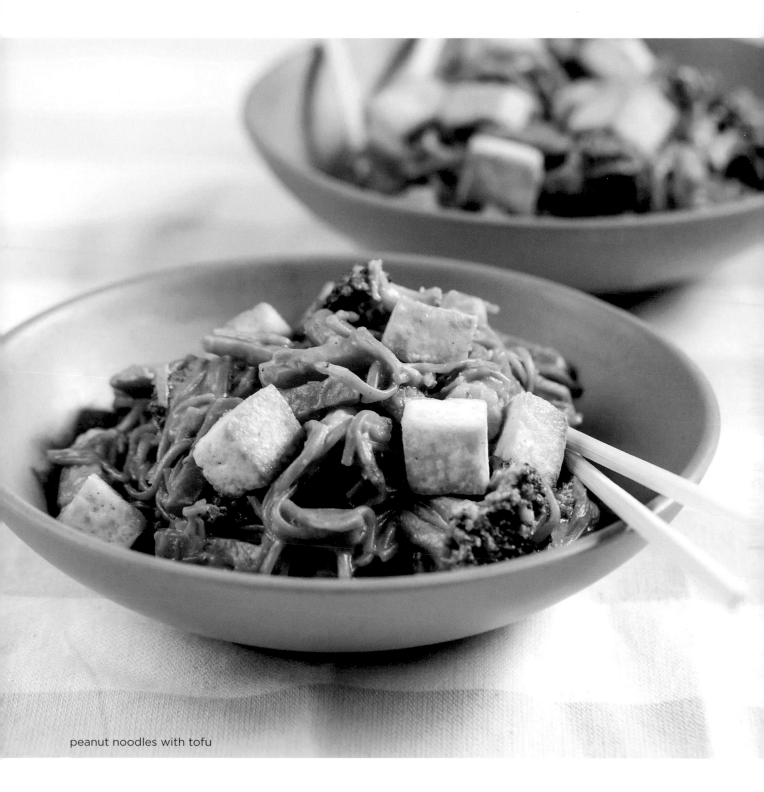

peanut noodles with tofu

tofu

dairy-free blueberry-banana pudding

total time: 5 minutes

1 (14-ounce) package of tofu

1¼ cup blueberries

1 banana, peeled

1 teaspoon vanilla

½ teaspoon agave nectar or honey

dollop of whipped cream (dairy free if you prefer)

Puree the tofu, 1 cup of blueberries, banana, vanilla, and sweetener in a blender until smooth.

Pour into two serving bowls and top with whipped cream and the remaining blueberries.

korean bbq tofu

preparation time: 10 minutes

marinating time: 30 minutes

cook time: 20 minutes

1 (16 ounce) package extra firm tofu

½ cup Korean bbq sauce

Slice the tofu into 12 long rectangles and lay out on paper towels. Place more paper towels on top. Press to remove excess moisture. (This will help to give the tofu some crunch.)

Place the tofu and ⅓ cup of marinade in a plastic container. Cover and refrigerate for 30 minutes or longer.

When you're ready to cook, preheat the oven to 400°F.

Cover a baking sheet with parchment paper and arrange the tofu slices in a single layer. Bake for 20–25 minutes until crispy, flipping halfway through. Coat with the remaining sauce, and serve with steamed veggies.

turkey

This traditional holiday bird is loaded with protein—there are about 24 grams in just 3 ounces—and B vitamins. It's also a good source of selenium, potassium, iron, and zinc. Though many of us don't think about eating turkey year-round, it is an excellent alternative to chicken, beef, or pork. The nutrients in turkey will also help your little munchkin build strong bones. It may also help boost immunity, prevent diabetes, and regulate stress and mood.

 Cook turkey breast until the meat is no longer pink and the internal temperature reaches 170°F.

turkey baby food

START WITH 2 thin-cut turkey breasts or ½ pound ground turkey

1. prep

Trim excess fat from turkey breasts.

2. cook

If using ground turkey, add the meat to a hot skillet and cook. Stir and break up the meat with a spatula until browned and cooked through, about 5–7 minutes. Drain any excess grease from the pan before serving. If using turkey breasts, choose from the following cooking methods.

SAUTÉ

cook time: 4 minutes

If using turkey breasts, heat the oil in a sauté pan over medium heat. Place the turkey fillets in the pan and cook until no longer pink, about 2–3 minutes on each side. Then chop.

BROIL

cook time: 10 minutes

Preheat the broiler to high. Cover a baking sheet with aluminum foil and spritz with cooking spray. Add the turkey cutlets to the pan and broil 5–8 minutes per side until cooked through. Chop when the turkey is cool enough to handle.

BAKE

cook time: 15 minutes

Preheat the oven to 350°F. Mist a baking dish with cooking spray. Add the turkey cutlets. Bake for 15–20 minutes or until cooked through, then chop.

3. add mix-ins & serve

simply turkey puree

6 months +

MIX-INS

¼ cup + 2 tablespoons breast milk, formula, or water

Place the cooked turkey and breast milk, formula, or water in a food processor until smooth and liquefied.

turkey with apples

7 months +

MIX-INS

1 apple

¼ cup + 2 tablespoons breast milk, formula, or water

Peel and quarter the apple, and then cook until tender (microwave for 2 minutes, boil for 10 minutes, steam for 12 minutes, or bake for 15 minutes at 375°F). Puree the apple and turkey, and breast milk, formula, or water in a food processor until smooth and soupy.

turkey with butternut squash

8 months +

MIX-INS

1½ cups fresh or frozen cubed butternut squash

⅓ cup tablespoons breast milk, formula, or water

Cook the butternut squash (microwave for 5–10 minutes or steam for 12 minutes). Puree turkey and squash, and breast milk, formula, or water until smooth.

turkey with green beans and prunes

9 months +

MIX-INS

¾ cup fresh green beans, ends cut off or frozen green beans

⅓ cup prunes

¼ cup breast milk, formula, or water

Bring a medium pot to a boil. Add the prunes and green beans and cook until the prunes are plump and the green beans are tender, about 3 minutes. Pour into a colander over the sink to drain. Puree the turkey, green beans, and prunes in a food processor with breast milk, formula, or water, and pulse to create a smooth puree with tiny lumps.

turkey, spinach, and sweet potatoes

10 months +

MIX-INS

1 small sweet potato

1 cup chopped frozen spinach

¼ cup + 1 tablespoon cup breast milk, formula, or water

Wash the potato, and then use a fork to poke holes all over the skin. Place on a microwave-safe dish, and microwave for 9 minutes, or until tender. Cut in half lengthwise and scoop the insides of the potato into a medium bowl. Cook the spinach as directed on the box. Then puree the turkey, spinach, sweet potatoes, and breast milk, formula, or water in a food processor to make a chunky puree.

meat and other proteins

turkey and sweet peas

11 months +

MIX-INS

¾ cup sweet peas

....

Cook the peas until tender (microwave, steam, or boil for 2–3 minutes). If using turkey fillets, cut into pea-sized cubes. Mix the turkey and peas together in a medium bowl. Serve a few pieces of turkey and peas at a time as finger food.

turkey with mixed vegetables

12 months +

MIX-INS

½ cup sweet corn kernels

3 baby carrots

....

Cook the corn and carrots until tender (microwave for 4 minutes, or steam or boil for 7 minutes).

Finely dice the carrots and turkey. Then mix some of the turkey, corn, and carrots together in a small bowl and serve as finger food.

mama recipes

lemon-rosemary turkey cutlets

preparation time: 5 minutes

cook time: 10 minutes

½ cup all-purpose flour

1 teaspoon dried rosemary

2 thin-cut turkey breast fillets

1 tablespoon canola oil

2 tablespoons lemon juice

....

Mix the flour and rosemary together in bowl. Rinse the turkey fillets under cold water. Then coat both sides in the flour mixture.

Heat the oil in a sauté pan over medium-high heat. Add the turkey and cook 2–3 minutes per side, or until cooked through. Sprinkle with lemon juice and serve with veggies.

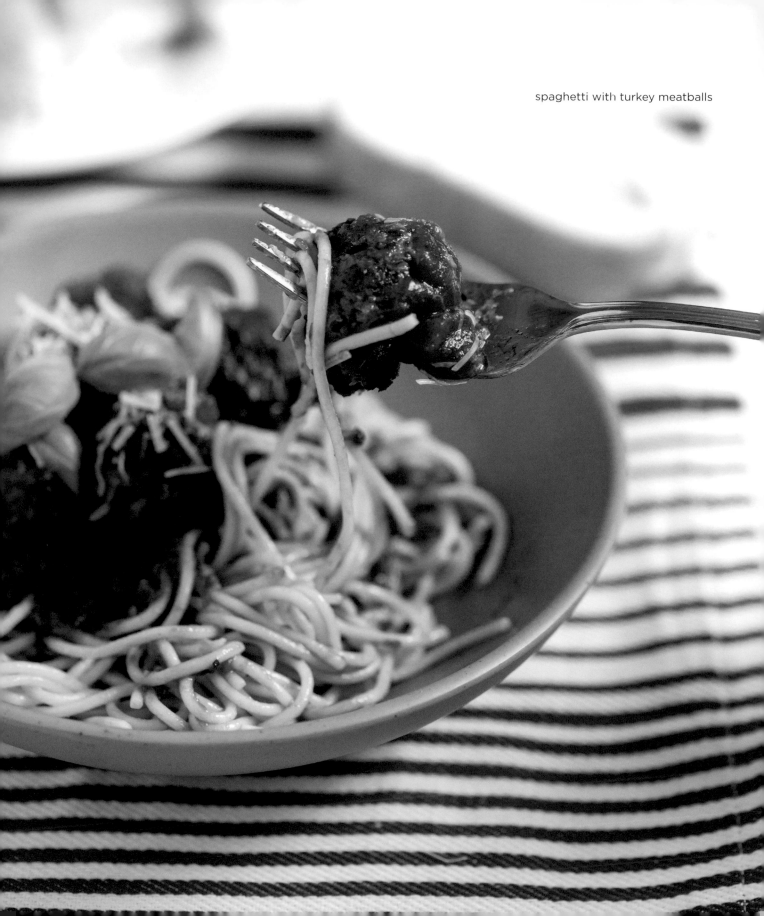

spaghetti with turkey meatballs

grilled turkey sandwich

preparation time: 10 minutes

cook time: 5 minutes

2 turkey fillets

1 tablespoon olive oil

2 ciabatta rolls

2 tablespoons mayonnaise

2 slices provolone cheese

2 lettuce leaves

2 slices tomato

Preheat the grill or grill pan to medium heat.

Season both sides of the turkey fillets with salt and pepper. Oil the grates of the hot grill with vegetable oil and place the turkey on the grill. Grill the cutlets until they are golden brown and cooked through, about 2–3 minutes per side.

Spread the top bun with mayo. Then layer the bottom half of each bun with turkey, cheese, lettuce, and tomato. Top with the other side of the bun.

spaghetti with turkey meatballs

preparation time: 15 minutes

cook time: 15 minutes

If you've never cooked with ground turkey before, this is the first recipe to try. I prefer these to beef meatballs because they're easier to make, healthier, and taste great. We almost always double this recipe and freeze the leftovers so that we have it on hand when we need a quick dinner.

½ pound spaghetti noodles

1 (24-ounce) jar of marinara sauce

1 pound ground turkey

½ cup breadcrumbs

1 tablespoon Italian seasoning

1 tablespoon ketchup

1 egg

½ cup onion, diced

2 garlic cloves, minced

¼ cup canola oil

Bring a large pot of water to a boil, and start heating the marinara sauce in a small saucepan over medium-low.

In a large bowl, combine the turkey, breadcrumbs, Italian seasoning, ketchup, egg, onion, and garlic. Roll the meat into 1-inch balls using your hands or a 1½-inch cookie scoop.

Heat the oil over medium-high heat in a large non-stick skillet. When the oil is hot, add the meatballs and cover. Turn them often to brown all sides. Reduce the heat to medium if the pan gets too hot. Cook for 8–12 minutes, or until the meatballs are cooked through. Then place on a paper towel–lined plate.

Cook the noodles according to the directions on the box, and then drain the water. Place the spaghetti onto serving plates. Top with meatballs and marinara sauce.

whole grains
and seeds

For babies who are six-to-eight months, you can make homemade infant cereal by grinding the grain into a powder. Then cook with water for a nice, smooth consistency. At around nine months, you may start to introduce baby to foods with a little texture, like small, soft lumps in purees. To get this consistency with grains, try cooking the whole grain, then pureeing it with breast milk, formula, or water until it reaches the right consistency for your baby.

barley

Barley is a nutritious ancient grain high in soluble and insoluble fiber. It is also a good source of selenium and niacin. These nutrients help to lower blood cholesterol levels, and may reduce risk of certain cancers, like breast and colon cancer. Barley is an excellent choice for nursing moms because it helps increase milk supply.

There are two main types of barley available—hulled and pearled barley. Hulled barley is the entire whole-grain kernel, so it contains more nutrients, but it takes longer to cook. Pearled barley, though still considered nutritious, is slightly processed (the husks are removed), but cooks quicker.

barley baby food

START WITH ¼ cup barley cereal or ½ cup hulled or pearled barley to add texture for babies 9 months +

For a complete guide on how to make your own infant cereal from whole grains, see page 242.

1. cook

To make barley infant cereal, bring 1 cup of water to a boil in a small saucepan. Reduce heat to low and slowly pour the barley infant cereal into the water as you stir with a whisk to prevent clumping. Keep stirring until the cereal is fully mixed into the water, about one minute. Cook for 20 minutes, until thickened, stirring occasionally.

To cook whole barley, place the barley and 1¼ cups of water (add an extra ¼ cup water for hulled barley) into a small saucepan and bring to a boil. Cover and reduce heat to a simmer. Cook pearled barley for 40 minutes, and hulled for up to an hour. Measure ¾ cup of cooked barley and store the rest in the refrigerator or freezer. Frozen barley is good for up to 3 months.

2. add mix-ins & serve

Serve on its own or with tasty mix-ins. If the cereal thickens before serving, add more liquid to make a creamy, soupy consistency.

simply barley cereal

7 months +

MIX-INS

3 tablespoons breast milk, formula, or water

Stir the breast milk, formula, or water into the barley cereal until smooth and soupy.

barley and butternut squash

8 months +

MIX-INS

¾ cup butternut squash, peeled and cubed

3 tablespoons breast milk, formula or water

Place the barley cereal in a medium bowl. Then add a few tablespoons of breast milk, formula, or water, and stir until creamy. Cook the squash until tender (microwave for 5–10 minutes, boil or steam for 12 minutes, or roast for 30 minutes at 400°F). Puree with 2 tablespoons of liquid until smooth. Swirl the squash puree into the cereal, or mix to combine.

barley and beef

9 months +

MIX-INS

1 small steak

¼ cup breast milk, formula, or water

Trim the steak, removing excess fat. Heat 2 teaspoons of oil in a sauté pan and add the beef. Sauté the steak until it's well-done, about 4 minutes per side. Let the steak rest for about 5 minutes, then slice, removing any excess fat. Whirl the beef and barley, and breast milk, formula, or water in a food processor to make a soft, lumpy puree.

barley, spinach, and cheese

10 months +

MIX-INS

2½ cups fresh spinach, washed

⅛ cup mozzarella cheese, grated

Cook the spinach until wilted (microwave for 2 minutes, steam or sauté for 2–5 minutes, or boil fo 3–5 minutes). Place the spinach, barley, and cheese in a food processor and blitz to create a chunky puree.

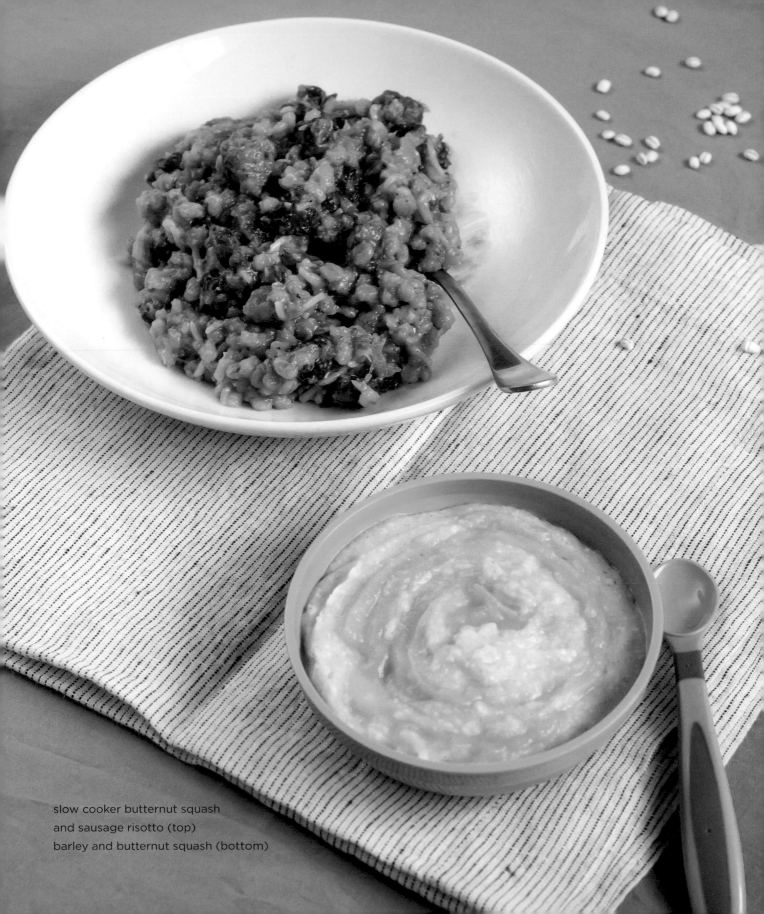

slow cooker butternut squash
and sausage risotto (top)
barley and butternut squash (bottom)

barley-millet porridge

11 months +

MIX-INS

¼ cup millet cereal

2 tablespoons breast milk, formula, or water

Bring ¾ cup of water to a boil in a small saucepan. Reduce heat to low. Slowly pour the millet infant cereal into the boiling water while stirring with a whisk to prevent clumping. Keep stirring until the cereal is fully mixed into the water, about one minute. Cook for 5 minutes, until thickened, stirring occasionally. Add the barley and breast milk, formula, or water. Stir to combine.

barley with oranges

12 months +

MIX-INS

2 orange slices

Look carefully at the orange slices, and remove any seeds and white strings. Finely dice the orange, and discard any tough pieces that might be difficult for baby to eat. Scoop a serving of barley into a small bowl and stir in the orange pieces.

mama recipes

orange and dark chocolate barley cereal

preparation time: 5 minutes

cook time: 35 minutes

¾ cup pearl barley

3 tablespoons low-fat milk

½ cup dark chocolate chips

1 orange, peeled and diced

Place the barley and 2 cups of water in a medium saucepan. Bring to a boil, then reduce heat to a simmer and cook uncovered for 35 minutes. Stir occasionally.

When the cereal is cooked, stir in the milk and chocolate chips. Top with diced oranges and serve.

slow cooker butternut squash and sausage risotto

preparation time: 15 minutes

slow-cook time: 3 hours

leftovers: 1 meal

1 tablespoon canola oil

1 lb. mild Italian sausage out of the casing

½ cup chopped white onion

1 cup pearled barley

3 cups chicken stock

2 cups butternut squash, peeled and diced

1 teaspoon dried sage

¾ cup grated Parmesan cheese

whole grains and seeds

Heat a nonstick skillet over medium heat. Then add the oil, onion, and sausage. Cook until the onion is tender and the sausage is browned.

Meanwhile, spray the slow cooker with cooking spray and add the barley, stock, squash, and sage. When the onion and sausage are finished cooking, add them to the slow cooker.

Cover and cook on high for 3 hours. Then stir in Parmesan cheese.

mushrooms and barley

preparation time: 10 minutes

cook time: 60 minutes

leftovers: 2 meals

½ cup white onions, diced

3 tablespoons olive oil

1 teaspoon dried thyme

1 cup sliced white mushrooms

1½ cup pearled barley

½ cup white wine

3½ cups vegetable stock

⅓ cup Parmesan cheese

In a large pot, heat the oil over medium heat. Then add the onions and thyme. Sauté until onions are nearly translucent, and add the mushrooms. Add another tablespoon of olive oil if the pan goes dry.

Once the mushrooms are cooked, add the barley and white wine. Stir constantly for 30 seconds, Add the vegetable stock and stir more. Bring to a boil, then cover and reduce heat to a simmer. Cook for 45 minutes, or until the barley is tender and the stock is absorbed. Season generously with salt and pepper.

Serve as a main dish or side. Top with cheese.

cheesy tomato and spinach barley

preparation: 5 minutes

cook time: 50 minutes

3 plum tomatoes

1¼ cups vegetable stock

¾ cup pearled barley

2 cloves of garlic, minced

2 cups fresh spinach, washed, and trimmed

1 teaspoon Italian seasoning

1 cup shredded mozzarella cheese

¼ cup fresh basil

In a medium pot, bring the whole tomatoes and stock to a boil. Then add the barley and garlic. Cover and simmer for 50 minutes, or until tender.

Add the spinach and Italian seasoning. Cover and cook for 2 minutes, or until the spinach is wilted. Remove from the heat and stir in the cheese and basil.

brown rice

Brown rice is packed full of nutrients, like fiber, protein, and vitamin B1. It helps increase milk production, boosts metabolism, and keeps you feeling full. Eating brown rice can also help protect from type 2 diabetes, heart disease, and cancer.

 White rice has very few nutritional benefits, since the healthy part of the grain gets removed when it's processed. Choose brown rice whenever possible, especially when cooking for baby.

brown rice baby food

START WITH ¼ cup brown rice cereal or ½ cup brown rice to add texture for babies 9 months +

1. cook

To make brown rice infant cereal, bring 1 cup of water to a boil in a small saucepan. Reduce heat to low, and slowly pour the rice infant cereal into the water while you stir with a whisk to prevent clumping. Keep stirring until the cereal is fully mixed into the water, about one minute. Cook for 15 minutes, until thickened, stirring occasionally.

To make brown rice, combine the rice and 1¾ cups water (add ¼ cup water if using short grain brown rice) in a small saucepan. Bring to a boil, then stir and bring to a simmer. Cover for 45 minutes, or until the rice is tender and the water has been absorbed.

2. add mix-ins & serve

Serve simply or with tasty mix-ins.

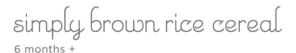

simply brown rice cereal
6 months +

MIX-INS

3 tablespoons breast milk, formula, or water

Stir breast milk, formula, or water into the cereal. As it sits, the cereal will thicken, absorbing the liquid. You may need to add more liquid just before serving so that it's a thin, soupy consistency.

prune-rice cereal
7 months +

MIX-INS

½ cup prunes

2 teaspoons breast milk, formula, or prune cooking water

Place the prunes in a small bowl and cover with boiling water. Let it sit until plump, about 3–5 minutes. Puree the prunes and stir into the rice cereal with the breast milk, formula, or cooking water.

apricot-brown rice cereal

8 months +

MIX-INS

½ cup dried apricots

Place the dried apricots in a microwave-safe dish. Then cover with water and cook for 2 minutes, or until plump. Puree the apricots, rice cereal, and 2 tablespoons of cooking water in a food processor until smooth and thick.

banana-asparagus rice cereal

9 months +

MIX-INS

1 banana, peeled

4 asparagus, trimmed

2 tablespoons breast milk, formula, or water

Cook the asparagus until tender (microwave for 2–4 minutes, steam or boil for 3–5 minutes, or roast for 15 minutes at 400°F). Puree the rice, banana, asparagus, and breast milk, formula, or water in a food processor to create a soft, chunky puree.

cauliflower and brown rice

10 months +

MIX-INS

1 cup cauliflower florets

¼ cup breast milk, formula, or water

Cook the cauliflower until tender (microwave 4–6 minutes, boil or steam for 25 minutes, or roasted for 25 minutes at 400°F). Place the cauliflower and rice, and breast milk, formula, or water in a food processor to create a chunky puree.

chicken and brown rice

11 months +

MIX-INS

1 small chicken breast

½ cup breast milk, formula, or water (optional)

Cook the chicken until no longer pink (sauté for 10 minutes, poach for 10 minutes, grill for 12 minutes, or bake for 15 minutes at 375°F). If using rice cereal, whirl the cereal and chicken, and breast milk, formula, or water in a food processor to make a chunky puree. If using whole rice, dice the chicken into pea-sized cubes. Then mix the rice and chicken together in a small bowl.

chinese rice bowl

12 months +

MIX-INS

½ cup frozen peas and carrots

Place the veggies in a microwave-safe bowl and add a tablespoon of water. Microwave for 2–3 minutes, or until heated through. Drain the water then stir into ½ cup of cooked rice. Place the remaining rice in a container and store in the refrigerator or freezer.

fluffy brown rice

total time: 45 minutes

You don't need a rice cooker to make fluffy rice at home. The trick? Use a wide skillet to help the rice cook evenly, and let it steam after it's finished cooking.

1 cup brown rice

1¾ cup water (for long grain rice) or 2 cups water (for short grain rice)

¼ teaspoon salt

1 tablespoon butter

In a large pot or wide skillet, add the rice, water, salt, and butter. Bring to a boil.

Cover, then reduce heat to a slow simmer. For chewy rice, cook for 30 minutes. For tender rice, cook for 50 minutes.

Turn off the burner and let it sit, covered and undisturbed, for 10 minutes. Fluff with a fork.

chicken fried rice

preparation time: 5 minutes

cook time: 45 minutes

¾ cup brown rice

5 tablespoons canola oil

3 eggs, beaten

1 chicken breast, sliced

½ cup white onion, diced

1½ cups frozen peas and carrots, thawed

¼ cup teriyaki sauce

In a medium saucepan, combine the rice and 1¼ cups water (for long grain rice) or 1½ cups water (for short grain rice). Bring to a boil, and then reduce heat to a simmer. Cover and cook for 40 minutes, or until tender.

When the rice has about 15 minutes left, line a plate with a paper towel and heat 2 tablespoons of oil in a large nonstick skillet over high heat. Swirl the oil so it coats the pan. Pour in the eggs, and let them cook (without touching them) for about 2 minutes, then flip. Once cooked, slide the eggs onto a plate and set aside.

Reduce the heat to medium-high and add the remaining oil to the pan. Add the chicken and cook halfway through. Then add the veggies. Cook until tender-crisp, about 5 minutes.

Reduce the heat to medium, and stir in the cooked rice, egg, and teriyaki sauce. Use a spatula to break up the egg and serve.

cardamom rice pudding

preparation time: 10 minutes

slow-cook time: 4 hours

leftovers: 2 servings

Cardamom is expensive. If you don't already have it in your pantry, use cinnamon instead. You can also swap brown raisins for the golden ones if that's what you have on hand.

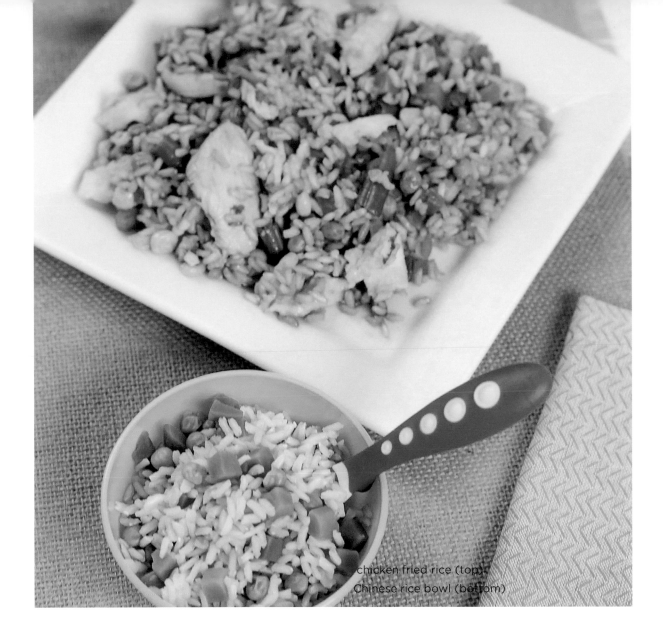

chicken fried rice (top)
Chinese rice bowl (bottom)

3 cups water

1 (13.5 ounce) can coconut milk

1½ cups milk

¾ cups brown rice

½ teaspoon cardamom

⅓ cup brown sugar

½ cup golden raisins

½ cup raw cashews or slivered almonds

Spray the slow-cooker with cooking spray. Then add the water, coconut milk, milk, rice, cardamom, and brown sugar. Stir to combine.

Cover and cook on high for 4 hours. Then stir in the golden raisins and nuts. The rice will continue to absorb the milk and will appear dry the next day, so stir in more milk before serving leftovers.

brown rice

buckwheat

Though used as a grain, buckwheat is actually the edible fruit seed from a plant related to rhubarb. It isn't at all related to wheat, and is gluten-free. Buckwheat is an excellent source of fiber, protein (23g in 1 cup), and magnesium. It contains all the essential amino acids, lowers cholesterol, promotes healthy blood sugar, and helps the body form strong bones and teeth.

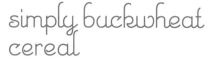 You'll likely find two types of whole buckwheat at the store—groats and kasha. Groats are uncooked buckwheat seeds, and kasha is roasted buckwheat. For a milder flavor, choose groats; kasha can taste strong and bitter.

buckwheat baby food

START WITH ¼ cup buckwheat infant cereal or ½ cup buckwheat groats to add texture for babies 9 months +

1. cook

For buckwheat infant cereal, bring 1 cup of water to a boil. Sprinkle in ¼ cup of ground buckwheat, whisking constantly. Continue to whisk occasionally for 10 minutes, or until thick and creamy.

For the buckwheat groats, combine 1 cup of water with the groats in a saucepan. Bring to a boil. Reduce the heat to a simmer and cover. Cook for 15–20 minutes, or until tender.

2. add mix-ins & serve

simply buckwheat cereal

8 months +

MIX-INS

2 tablespoons breast milk, formula, or water

Stir the breast milk, formula, or water into the buckwheat cereal until smooth and creamy.

whole grains and seeds

chickpea, kale, and buckwheat puree

10 months +

MIX-INS

¼ cup cooked chickpeas

¼ cup kale, chopped

2 tablespoons breast milk, formula, or water

Cook the kale until wilted (microwave for 1–2 minutes, or sauté for 5 minutes). Place the buckwheat, chickpeas, kale, and breast milk, formula, or water in a food processor and blitz to create a soft, lumpy puree.

blueberry-banana buckwheat

10 months +

MIX-INS

1 cup blueberries, washed

1 small banana

2 tablespoons breast milk, formula, or water

Use a fork to mash the blueberries and bananas together, or pulse in a food processor, leaving some small lumps. In a medium bowl, stir the buckwheat and mashed fruit, and breast milk, formula, or water together until combined.

cheesy buckwheat

11 months +

MIX-INS

½ cup shredded Swiss cheese

2 tablespoons breast milk, formula, or water

If using whole buckwheat, place the cheese and cooked buckwheat, and breast milk, formula, or water in a food processor and pulse to create a course and chunky puree. If using buckwheat cereal, stir the cheese and breast milk, formula, or water into the cereal until combined.

strawberry-buckwheat cereal

12 months +

MIX-INS

¼ cup strawberries, finely diced

2 tablespoons breast milk, formula, or water

In a small bowl, add a portion of buckwheat cereal. Then stir in the strawberries and breast milk, formula, or water.

mushroom and swiss buckwheat crepes

preparation time: 10 minutes

cook time: 15 minutes

Crepes are often thought of as hard to make, but these ones are foolproof. Just make a thin pancake and add toppings inside like an omelet, and it's done!

¼ **cup all-purpose flour**

¼ **cup ground buckwheat**

1 **egg**

¼ **cup milk**

¼ **cup water**

1 **tablespoon sugar**

1½ **cups sliced white mushrooms**

1½ **tablespoons butter**

1 **cup shredded Swiss cheese**

In a medium bowl, whisk together the flour, ground buckwheat, egg, milk, water, and sugar.

Melt 1 tablespoon of butter in a nonstick skillet over medium-high heat. Then add the mushrooms. Season with salt and pepper and sauté until tender, about 5 minutes. Pour into a small bowl and cover to keep warm.

Wipe the pan with a paper towel, and melt the rest of the butter over medium heat. Pour the crepe batter into a 2-cup measuring device. Then pour half of the crepe batter into the pan. Swirl to make a thin pancake that takes up the whole pan.

When the edges are dry and start to pull away from the sides, flip the crepe. Arrange half of the cheese and mushrooms along the center and fold. Use a spatula to transfer the crepe to a plate. Then use the rest of the ingredients make the other crepe.

chocolate-buckwheat mug cake

preparation time: 10 minutes

cook time: 2 minutes

serves: 1

This is the perfect morning boost after a long sleepless night. It's high in protein, fiber, and iron, and will prepare you for your day. Keep the dry mix on hand for easy preparation.

½ **banana**

¼ **cup ground buckwheat**

1 **tablespoon buckwheat groats**

2 **tablespoons Mexican hot chocolate powder (or hot chocolate mix)**

¼ **teaspoon baking powder**

1 **tablespoon milk**

1 **egg white**

fruit for topping

Butter a large mug. In a medium bowl, mash the banana with a fork until smooth. Stir in the ground buckwheat, groats, hot chocolate powder, baking powder, milk, and egg white.

Pour the batter into the mug and microwave for 90 seconds. Top with fresh fruit, like blueberries and sliced bananas.

cream of buckwheat with strawberries

preparation time: 5 minutes

cook time: 5 minutes

1 cup low-fat milk

½ cup ground buckwheat

½ cup strawberries, sliced

In a medium saucepan, combine the milk and 1 cup of water. Heat until almost boiling. Then move the saucepan off the burner and whisk in the ground buckwheat.

Reduce heat to low, and return the pan to the burner. Stir constantly for about one minute, until thick. Then pour into two bowls and top with sliced strawberries.

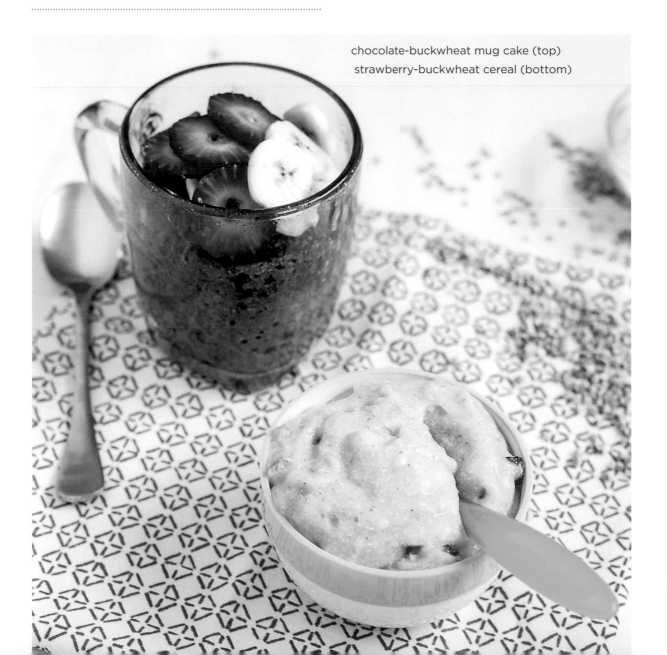

chocolate-buckwheat mug cake (top)
strawberry-buckwheat cereal (bottom)

213

bulgur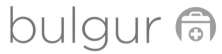

Bulgur (also known as bulgur wheat or cracked bulgur) is created from pre-cooked, crushed wheat berries. It is extremely easy to cook, packed with protein, and contains even more fiber than brown rice (17 grams of protein and 26 grams of fiber in just one cup!). Bulgur may also help protect against heart disease and certain cancers, like colon cancer. The body also digests bulgur slowly so it will keep you feeling nourished and full.

bulgur baby food

START WITH ⅓ cup bulgur cereal or ⅓ cup coarse bulgur to add texture for babies 9 months +

1. cook

To cook bulgur infant cereal, bring 1¼ cups of water to a boil. Reduce the heat to low, and slowly pour the cereal into the boiling water while stirring with a whisk to prevent clumping. Keep stirring until the cereal is fully mixed into the water, about one minute. Cook for 7 minutes, stirring occasionally.

To cook bulgur, bring ⅔ cup of water to a boil. Stir in the bulgur. Turn off the heat and let the bulgur soak for 15–20 minutes, or until tender. Then drain any excess water.

2. add mix-ins & serve

Serve on its own or with tasty mix-ins.

simply bulgur cereal
8 months +

MIX-INS

2 tablespoons breast milk, formula, or water

Stir breast milk, formula, or water into bulgur cereal until smooth and creamy. Add more liquid if the cereal thickens before serving.

peach-bulgur puree

9 months +

MIX-INS

1 peach

2 tablespoons breast milk, formula, or water

Cut the peach in half and remove the pit. Cook the peach until tender (microwave for 2 minutes, steam for 5 minutes, or roast for 20 minutes at 425°F). When cool to the touch, slice or peel off the skin. Puree the bulgur and peach, and breast milk, formula, or water in a food processor until smooth with some tiny lumps.

bulgur-raisin cereal

10 months +

MIX-INS

¼ cup raisins

2 tablespoons breast milk, formula, or raisin cooking water

Place the raisins in a bowl and cover with hot water. Let the raisins sit for 5 minutes, or until plump. Pulse the bulgur and raisins, and breast milk, formula, or water in a food processor until coarse and chunky.

bulgur-lentil salad

11 months +

MIX-INS

¼ cup green lentils

Place the lentils in a strainer and rinse under cool water. Pick out any debris or shriveled lentils. Cook the lentils with 1 cup of water (microwave uncovered for 15 minutes or simmer for 25 minutes on the stove) until tender. Roughly mash the bulgur and lentils until combined.

corn and bulgur salad

12 months +

MIX-INS

⅔ cup frozen corn kernels

Cook the corn according to the directions on the package. In a small bowl, mix the bulgur and corn together. Serve as finger food.

microwave bulgur pilaf

total time: 20 minutes

½ cup bulgur

1 cup chicken stock

2 tablespoons butter

½ teaspoon salt

⅛ teaspoon onion powder

Stir all of the ingredients together in a large microwave-safe bowl. Microwave for 4 minutes, and then let stand for 15 minutes to finish cooking. Fluff before serving.

raisin-cookie porridge

total time: 20 minutes

½ cup medium-grind bulgur

¼ teaspoon salt

⅓ cup low-fat milk

2 tablespoons brown sugar

⅓ cup raisins

½ tablespoon cinnamon

¼ teaspoon vanilla extract

Place the bulgur, cup of water, and salt in a medium saucepan. Bring to a boil, and then cover and simmer for 10–15 minutes, or until tender. Stir in the remaining ingredients and serve warm.

quickie tabbouleh salad

total time: 20 minutes

½ cup bulgur wheat

1 cup cherry tomatoes, halved

½ cup crumbled feta or goat cheese

½ cup fresh parsley, chopped

2 tablespoons lemon juice

Bring 1 cup of water to a boil in a small saucepan. Turn off the heat and add the bulgur. Cover and soak for 15–20 minutes, until tender. Meanwhile, prepare the tomatoes and parsley.

Drain the bulgur and place in a large bowl. Add the tomatoes, cheese, and parsley. Season to taste with salt and pepper.

chia seeds

Chia (cousin to the famous ch-ch-ch-chia plant pet) is a nutritious seed that helps boost energy and endurance. Known as a super-seed in the diet and fitness world, chia seeds contain more Omega-3 fatty acids than salmon, and are high in fiber and protein. Chia also promotes a healthy brain, heart, teeth, and bones.

Dried chia seeds are small and crunchy, and can be added into yogurt, smoothies, drinks, muffins, and salads. When soaked, chia absorbs liquid and plumps like tapioca pearls, making a gel or thick and creamy pudding, depending on the liquid.

Chia seeds are fully digestible whole, but some nutritionists suggest grinding them for baby. If you grind chia seeds, use them right away since they don't stay fresh for long.

Though super nutritious, only serve chia to baby a few times a week in small batches. Consider it a nutritional booster for other foods, not the main ingredient for your child's meal. Too much chia at one time can cause constipation or bloating.

baby food with chia seeds

START WITH 2 teaspoons ground chia or 2 teaspoons whole chia seeds

1. prep

To make ground chia, pour chia seeds in a coffee or spice grinder and grind into a fine powder.

2. add mix-ins & serve

Stir chia into fruit purees or yogurt. Serve them crunchy or plump.

pear-plum chia
9 months +

MIX-INS

1 pear, peeled, halved, and cored

2 plums, halved and cored

¼ cup breast milk, formula or water (optional)

Cook the fruit until soft (microwave for 5 minutes or heat in a saucepan for 25 minutes). Then remove the plum peel. Blend the pear and plum together until smooth with tiny lumps. Stir in chia seeds, and serve or pour into a lidded container and refrigerate for five or more hours.

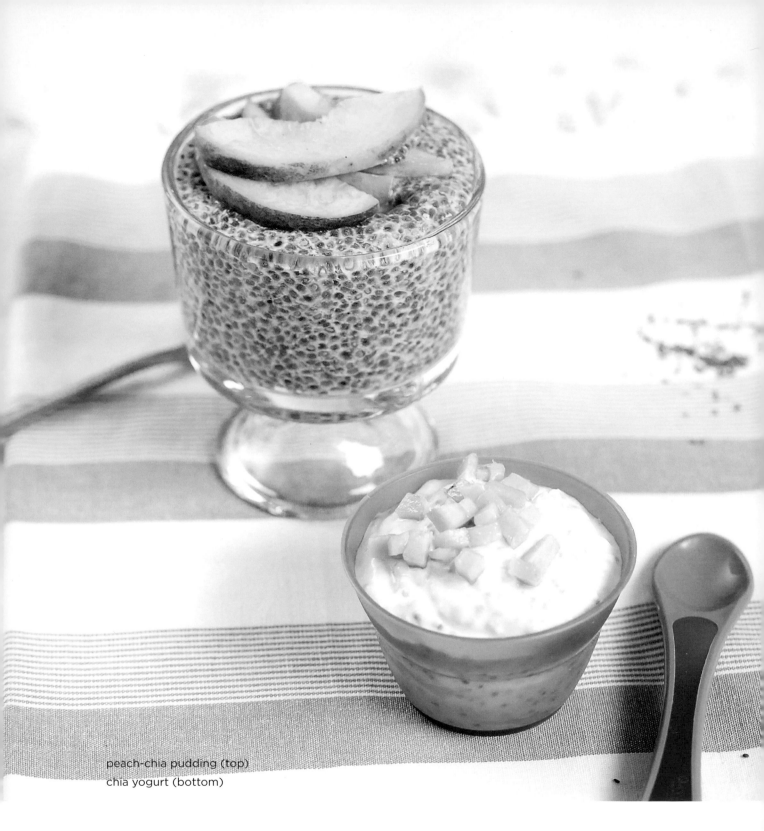

peach-chia pudding (top)
chia yogurt (bottom)

218

whole grains and seeds

peach chia

10 months +

MIX-INS

2 peaches

2 tablespoons breast milk, formula, or water

Cut the peach in half and remove the pit. Cook the peach until tender (microwave for 2 minutes, steam for 5 minutes, or roast for 20 minutes at 425°F). When the peach is cool, peel off the skin. Puree the peach until smooth, and then stir in the chia. Cover and refrigerate for five or more hours until the chia is plump. Just before serving, stir in the breast milk, formula, or water.

chia yogurt

11 months +

MIX-INS

½ cup plain, full-fat yogurt

1 tablespoon chia seeds

Stir the yogurt and chia together in a small bowl. Serve immediately or cover and refrigerate until the chia is plump.

raspberry chia

12 months +

MIX-INS

1 cup raspberries

Place the raspberries in a small saucepan, and cook over medium heat until broken down into a sauce. Pour the raspberry puree into a fine mesh sieve set over a bowl to strain out the seeds. Stir the chia into the raspberry puree. Once cooled, cover and place in the refrigerator until the chia is plump.

mama recipes

peach-chia pudding

preparation time: 5 minutes

wait time: 5½ hours

My sister-in-law introduced me to chia a few years ago when she made a similar chia pudding recipe for a family holiday. Let's just say we all cleaned our bowls. This is my take on the popular no-cook chia pudding.

1¼ cup vanilla almond milk

¼ cup chia seeds

1 teaspoon almond extract

1 peach, diced

In a lidded container, stir together 1 cup of almond milk, chia, and almond extract. Cover, then place in the refrigerator for 5 hours or overnight. If you can, stir after 2 hours to loosen the chia.

Stir in the remaining ¼ cup of almond milk and the diced peaches. Spoon into two bowls, or keep it all for yourself and it eat right out of the container.

chocolate-chia pudding

preparation time: 5 minutes

wait time: 4 hours

If you love chocolate pudding, you'll love this version. It's super easy to make, and it tastes indulgent even though it's not. For even more of a flavor pop,
top with sliced strawberries.

1¼ cups chocolate almond milk

¼ cup chia seeds

1 tablespoon ground flax seed

1 teaspoon vanilla extract

Stir all of the ingredients together in a lidded container. Then cover and refrigerate for 4 hours or overnight. Use a spoon to stir before serving.

strawberry-lemon chia water

preparation time: 3 minutes

wait time: 10 minutes

Who says water has to be boring? With just a little fruit and chia you can have yourself a bright and flavorful energy drink.

2 cups water

1 tablespoon chia seeds

½ lemon, sliced

½ cup strawberries, sliced

Pour the water into a large glass or 16-ounce water bottle. Then add the chia, strawberries, and lemon slices. Stir or shake to combine.

Refrigerate (minimum of 10 minutes, maximum overnight) to allow the chia to plump and the fruit to infuse into the water. The longer it sits the more flavorful the mixture will be. Remove the fruit, or keep it—whichever you prefer!

whole grains and seeds

flaxseed

Flaxseed is an excellent source of fiber and Omega-3 fatty acids. Flax has been found to relieve depression and constipation, boost sex drive, lower blood pressure, and regulate menstrual cycles. It may also protect against heart disease, as well as breast, colon, and prostate cancers.

To get all of the nutritional benefits of flaxseed, be sure to grind it first. Otherwise the small seed will pass through you (and baby) undigested. If you grind your own flax, use it within 24 hours. You can also buy pre-ground flaxseed that's packaged to help it last longer.

Just like chia, only serve flaxseed a few times a week in small batches. Consider it a nutritional booster for other foods, not the main ingredient for your child's meal.

baby food with flaxseed

START WITH ½ teaspoon ground flaxseed

1. prep

Place flaxseed in a food processor or spice grinder, and grind into a fine powder.

2. add mix-ins & serve

Add ground flax to prepared cereal, yogurt, cottage cheese, purees, smoothies and more.

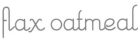

flax oatmeal

10 months +

MIX-INS

¼ cup quick-cooking, steel cut oats

2 tablespoons breast milk, formula, or water

Bring ¾ cup of water to a boil. Reduce heat to low, and then stir in oats. Cook uncovered for 5–8 minutes, or until tender. Stir in the flaxseed and breast milk, formula, or water to make a soft, lumpy oatmeal.

flax cottage cheese

11 months +

MIX-INS

½ cup full-fat cottage cheese

In a small bowl, stir the cottage cheese and flax until combined.

berry-banana yogurt with flax

12 months +

MIX-INS

½ banana

½ cup frozen mixed berries

½ cup plain full-fat yogurt

Blend the banana, berries, yogurt, and flax together until smooth.

mama recipes

berry-flax smoothie

total time: 5 minutes

2 cups frozen mixed berries

1 cup spinach, washed

1 banana, peeled

1 cup milk

1 tablespoon flaxseed meal

Place all of the ingredients in a blender and puree until smooth.

cherry-granola crisp

preparation time: 10 minutes

cook time: 35 minutes

2 cups frozen cherries

1 tablespoon flour

¼ cup sugar

1 cup granola (recommended: granola with pecans)

2 tablespoons ground flax

3 tablespoons melted butter

Preheat the oven to 375°F and butter a 2-cup baking dish or 9 × 5 × 4-inch loaf pan.

Place the cherries in the baking dish and toss with the flour and sugar. Combine the granola, ground flax, and melted butter, and sprinkle over the cherries.

Bake for 35 minutes, until the top is golden brown and the filling is bubbly. Serve warm with whipped cream or vanilla ice cream, or serve cool for breakfast with yogurt.

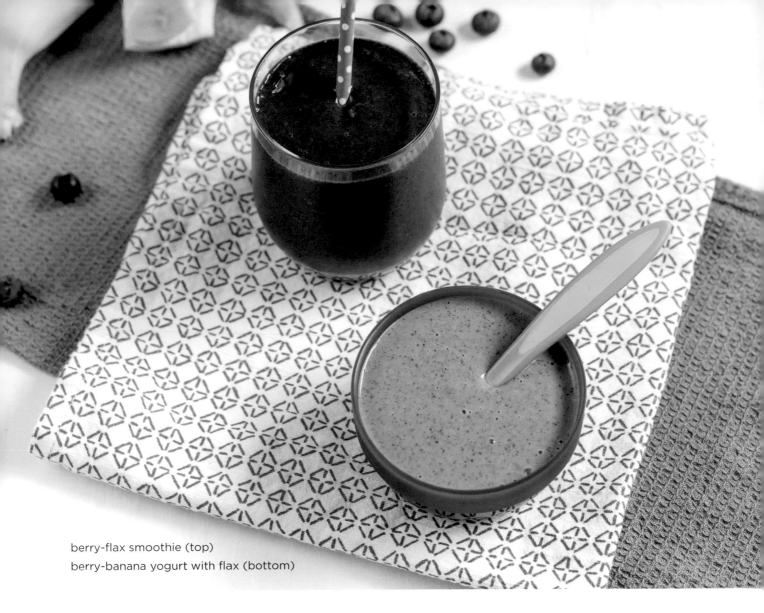

berry-flax smoothie (top)
berry-banana yogurt with flax (bottom)

cottage cheese with fruit, flax, and nuts

preparation time: 5 minutes

2 cups cottage cheese

1 teaspoons ground flaxseed

½ cup fresh fruit (like strawberries or blackberries)

¼ cup nuts (like pecans or cashews)

Scoop the cottage cheese into a two bowls. Top with flax, fruit, and nuts.

millet

Millet is an easily digestible, gluten-free seed that's a staple in many African and Asian cultures. It contains healthy doses of protein, magnesium, and antioxidants, and helps regulate blood pressure, cholesterol, and blood sugar. Millet promotes healthy muscles, bones, hair, and nerves, and may even soothe migraine and asthma symptoms.

millet baby food

START WITH ¼ cup millet cereal or ¼ cup millet to add texture for babies 9 months +

1. cook

To make millet cereal, bring 1 cup of water to a boil in a small saucepan. Reduce the heat to low, and then slowly pour the cereal into the boiling water. Mix well and cook for 10 minutes, stirring often until thickened.

To make millet, combine ¾ cup of water with the millet in a saucepan. Bring to a boil, and then cover and reduce heat to a simmer until all of the liquid absorbs, about 20 minutes. Move the pot off the burner. Cover for 10 minutes to steam until tender.

2. add mix-ins & serve

Serve simply or with tasty mix-ins.

simply millet cereal
7 months +

MIX-INS

⅓ cup breast milk, formula, or water

Stir the breast milk, formula, or water into the millet cereal to make a creamy, soupy consistency. Add a little more liquid just before serving if the cereal thickens.

brown rice and millet porridge
8 months +

MIX-INS

¼ cup brown rice

¼ cup breast milk, formula, or water

Bring the rice and ¾ cup of water to a boil. Stir, then cover and simmer for 45 minutes, or until the rice is tender and the water absorbed. Place the brown rice and millet, and breast milk, formula, or water in a food processor and pulse to create a soft, lumpy puree.

pumpkin-millet cereal

9 months +

MIX-INS

½ cup peeled and cubed pumpkin

¼ cup breast milk, formula, or water

....

Cook the cubed pumpkin until tender (microwave for 5–10 minutes, boil or steam for 12 minutes, or roast for 30 minutes at 400°F). Puree the pumpkin and breast milk, formula, or water in a food processor until smooth. Then stir into cereal until combined.

fig-millet porridge

10 months +

If you can't find fresh figs, fresh apricots are also delicious in this recipe!

MIX-INS

2 fresh figs

¼ cup breast milk, formula, or water

....

Cut off the stems from the figs and halve. Blitz the figs and breast milk, formula, or water in a food processor to make a lumpy puree. Then stir into millet.

cheesy brussels sprout millet

11 months +

MIX-INS

½ cup brussels sprouts

3 tablespoons shredded cheddar cheese

1 tablespoon breast milk, formula, or water

....

Slice off the stems of the sprouts and remove the outer leaves. Cook the brussels sprouts until tender (microwave for 2 minutes, boil or steam for 5–10 minutes, or roast for 20 minutes at 400°F).

Pulse the brussels sprouts and breast milk, formula, or water in a food processor to finely chop. Then transfer to a bowl and stir in cheese.

pineapple millet

12 months +

MIX-INS

¼ cup pineapple, finely diced

....

In a small bowl, stir the pineapple and millet together until combined.

pineapple and millet cereal

total time: 35 minutes

1 cup millet

¼ cup milk

¾ cup pineapple

2 tablespoons honey

Combine the millet and 2½ cups water in a medium saucepan and bring to a boil. Cover and simmer for 20 minutes, or until the millet is puffed up and tender, and the liquid absorbed.

Shut off the burner, and then stir in the milk. Cover and let sit for 10 minutes to steam. Pour the millet cereal into two bowls. Top with pineapple and drizzle with honey.

cheddar millet with roasted brussels sprouts

preparation time: 10 minutes

cook time: 30 minutes

leftovers: 2 servings

½ pound brussels sprouts, trimmed and halved

2 tablespoons olive oil

2¼ cups chicken stock

¾ cup millet

1 garlic clove, minced

1 cup shredded cheddar cheese

Preheat oven to 400°F. Toss the brussels sprouts in about a tablespoon of oil, and spread on the baking sheet in a single layer. Season with salt and pepper. Roast for 20 minutes, flipping halfway through.

Meanwhile, pour the chicken stock into a medium saucepan and bring to a boil. Heat a skillet over medium-high heat. Add the remaining tablespoon of oil, and the millet and garlic to the skillet. Cook to toast the millet, about 2 minutes. Then pour the millet into the saucepan with the stock.

Cover and simmer for 20 minutes. Then shut off the heat and stir in the brussels sprouts and cheese. Cover and let sit 10 minutes more. Stir and fluff with a fork.

millet and mushroom pilaf

preparation: 10 minutes

cook time: 35 minutes

1 cup millet

2 tablespoons olive oil

½ cup diced white onion

¾ cup sliced white mushrooms

1 tablespoon dried parsley

Combine the millet and 2½ cups of water in a medium saucepan and bring to a boil. Cover and simmer until all of the water has been absorbed, about 25 minutes. Then shut off the heat, and let sit, covered for 10 minutes to steam.

Meanwhile, heat the olive oil in a nonstick skillet. Add the onions and mushrooms to the pan and sauté until tender, about 5 minutes.

Stir the millet and parsley into the mushroom mixture, and stir to combine. Season with salt and pepper and fluff with a fork.

oats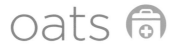

Oats are extremely good for your heart, and a good source of soluble and insoluble fiber and B vitamins. They also help increase milk supply for those nursing moms. Oatmeal makes an awesome breakfast because it's digested slowly, so it'll keep you feeling full and energized through the morning.

oat baby food

START WITH ½ cup oat cereal, or ½ cup rolled or quick-cooking steel cut oats to add texture for babies 9 months +

1. cook

To make oat infant cereal, bring 2 cups of water to a boil in a small saucepan. Reduce heat to low and slowly pour the cereal into the water. Mix well and cook for 20 minutes, stirring often until thickened.

To make oatmeal bring water (¾ cup for rolled or 1½ cups for steel-cut oats) to a boil in a small saucepan. Add oats, and then reduce heat to low and simmer uncovered for 5–7 minutes.

2. add mix-ins & serve

simply oats baby cereal
6 months +

MIX-INS
1 tablespoon breast milk, formula, or water

Stir breast milk, formula, or water into oat infant cereal to create a smooth and soupy consistency. Add more liquid if the cereal thickens before serving.

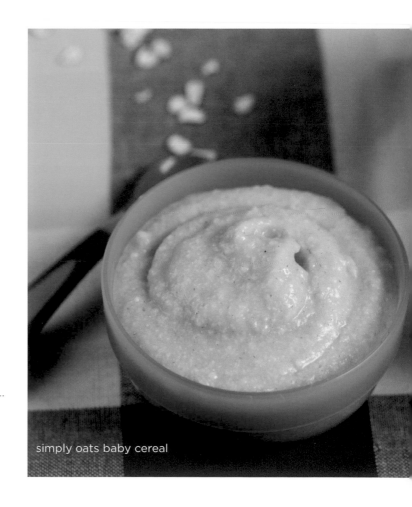

simply oats baby cereal

oat and brown rice cereal

7 months +

MIX-INS

¼ cup brown rice infant cereal

¼ cup breast milk, formula, or water

Bring 1 cup of water to a boil. Then reduce heat to low, and slowly pour in the ground brown rice. Mix well and cook for 15 minutes, or until thickened. Stir in the oat cereal and breast milk, formula, or water to make a smooth, creamy cereal.

pear oatmeal

8 months +

MIX-INS

1 pear

Wash and peel the pear. Cut it in half and remove the core and seeds. Cook the pear (microwave for 2 minutes, steam for 3–5 minutes, or roast for 15 minutes at 425°F). Puree the pear until smooth, and then stir into the oat cereal.

carrots and oats

9 months +

MIX-INS

½ cup baby carrots

3 tablespoons breast milk, formula, or water

Place the carrots in a microwave-safe dish with a splash of water. Microwave for 3–6 minutes, or until tender. Then drain the water. Place the carrots in a food processor to finely dice. Then stir into cereal with the breast milk, formula, or water.

plum-banana oatmeal

10 months +

MIX-INS

1 plum

½ banana, peeled

Place the plum in a saucepan and cover with water. Bring to a boil and simmer for 5 minutes, or until tender. Let cool slightly, then halve, pit, and peel. Place the plum, banana, and oats in a food processor to form a lumpy puree.

oat and quinoa hot cereal

11 months +

MIX-INS

½ cup quinoa cereal

3 tablespoons breast milk, formula, or water

To cook quinoa, combine 1½ cups of water with the quinoa in a saucepan. Bring to a boil, cover, and reduce heat to low. Cook until most of the water has been absorbed, about 12 minutes. Stir in the cooked oats and breast milk, formula, or water.

oatmeal with flax and fruit

12 months +

MIX-INS

2 tablespoons breast milk, formula, or water

⅛ cup strawberries or blueberries, finely diced

ground flaxseed

Stir the breast milk, formula, or water into the oatmeal. Then scoop a serving into a baby bowl. Stir in some fruit and a tiny sprinkle of flaxseed.

muesli

preparation time: 10 minutes

wait time: 8 hours

This is one of the easiest breakfasts I make. We have it about once a week in our house. When berries are out of season in the winter, I leave them out and get added flavor from cream top yogurt instead.

1 cup vanilla yogurt

1 cup rolled oats

½ cup milk

1 cup mixed fruit (blueberries and sliced strawberries work well)

Stir the ingredients together. Then cover and refrigerate overnight. The oats will absorb the liquid and become tender by morning. Stir in an extra splash of milk just before serving.

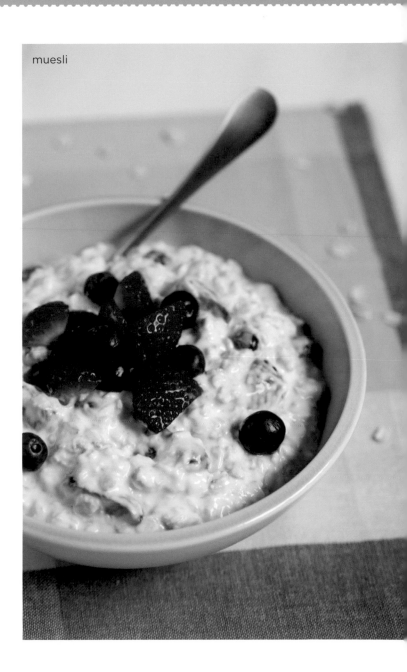

muesli

oats

oatmeal with caramelized pears

preparation time: 5 minutes

cook time: 15 minutes

2 tablespoons butter

1 pear, diced

2 tablespoons brown sugar

1 cup rolled oats

1 cup milk

Heat the butter over medium heat in a nonstick skillet. Add the diced pears and cook until tender. Then sprinkle with brown sugar. Cook until the pears are caramelized in brown sugar.

Meanwhile, bring the oats, milk, and one cup of water to a boil over medium-high heat. Reduce heat to a simmer and cook until oats are tender, about 5 minutes.

Scoop the oatmeal into two serving bowls, then top with caramelized pears.

slow cooker steel-cut oats

preparation time: 5 minutes

slow-cook time: 7 hours

You can make this recipe your own by adding diced fruit, dried fruit, spices, or nuts to the oats before or after cooking.

6 cups water

½ cups steel-cut oats

¼ teaspoon salt

½ cup milk

Place the water, oats, and salt in a slow-cooker. Cover and cook on low for 7 hours.

In the morning, stir in milk until creamy. Then top with your favorite oatmeal toppings.

whole grains and seeds

quinoa

Quinoa is the gluten-free seed from the quinoa plant. It is one of the best sources of protein, containing all nine amino acids (usually only present in animal-based protein sources like beef). It is also extremely high in fiber, manganese, magnesium, and riboflavin. Quinoa is good for your heart and brain and helps your body build strong bones and teeth. It may even boost your energy and alleviate migraine and anxiety symptoms.

quinoa baby food

START WITH ¼ cup quinoa cereal or ½ cup quinoa to add texture for babies 9 months +

1. prep

If making whole quinoa, rinse well with water.

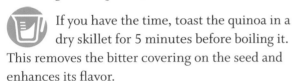 If you have the time, toast the quinoa in a dry skillet for 5 minutes before boiling it. This removes the bitter covering on the seed and enhances its flavor.

2. cook

To cook quinoa infant cereal, bring ¾ cups of water to a boil in a small saucepan. Reduce heat to low and slowly pour the ground quinoa into the boiling water. Mix well. Cook for 12 minutes, stirring often until thickened.

To cook whole quinoa, combine 1¼ cups of water with the quinoa in a saucepan and bring to a boil. Cover, reduce heat to medium-low, and cook until most of the water has been absorbed, about 15 minutes. Turn off the heat, and let the quinoa steam for 5 minutes. Fluff with a fork.

3. add mix-ins & serve

Serve on its own or with tasty mix-ins.

simply quinoa infant cereal

8 months +

MIX-INS

2 tablespoons breast milk, formula, or water

Stir breast milk, formula, or water into cooked quinoa cereal to create a smooth, soupy consistency. Add more liquid just before serving if the cereal thickens.

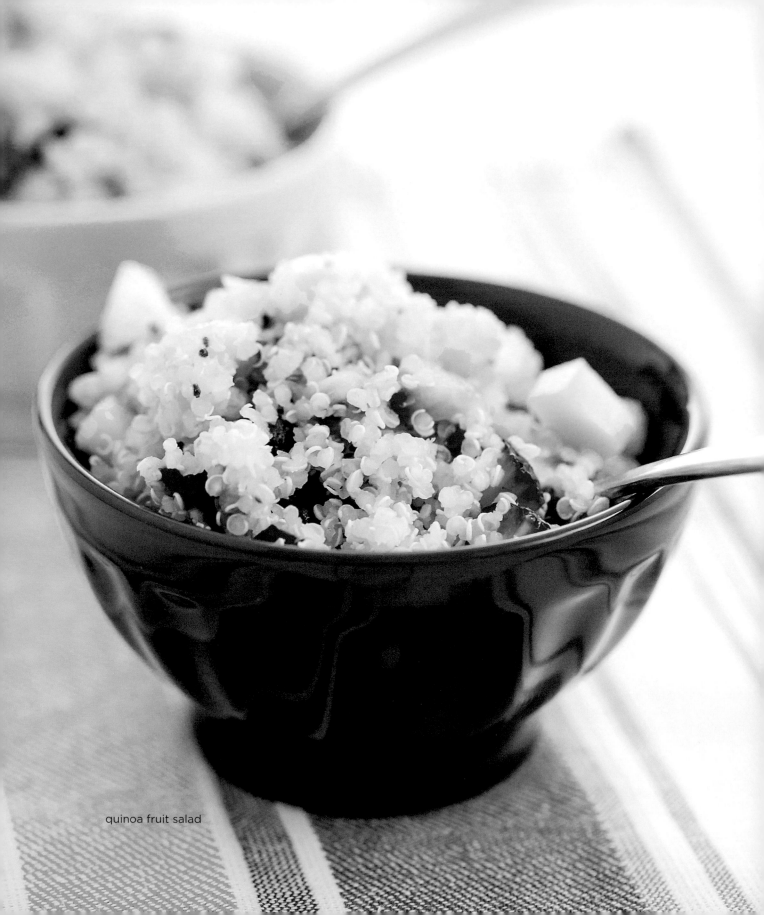

quinoa fruit salad

plum-yogurt quinoa

9 months +

MIX-INS

1 plum

¼ cup full-fat yogurt

Cool the quinoa to room temperature. Meanwhile, halve the plums and remove the pit and peel. Place the plum halves in a microwave-safe dish with a splash of water. Microwave for 2–3 minutes until tender. Place the cooled quinoa, plums, and yogurt in a food processor and puree to create a soft-mashed puree.

three-grain oatmeal

10 months +

MIX-INS

¼ cup rolled oats

¼ teaspoon ground flaxseed

2 tablespoons breast milk, formula, or water

Bring ½ cup of water to a boil in a small sauce-pan, and add the oats. Reduce heat and simmer, uncovered, for 5 minutes. Let the oatmeal cool. Combine all of the ingredients in a food processor. Pulse 2–3 times to make a chunky oatmeal.

edamame-kale quinoa

11 months +

MIX-INS

½ cup frozen, shelled edamame

½ cup chopped kale

2 tablespoons breast milk, formula, or water

Cook the edamame (microwave for 1–2 minutes or boil for 5 minutes). Add the kale and cook until wilted. Place ½ the quinoa, edamame, kale, and breast milk, formula, or water in a food processor and pulse to create a chunky puree.

peach quinoa

12 months +

MIX-INS

1 peach, halved

Cook the peach until tender (microwave for 2 minutes, steam for 5 minutes, or roast for 20 minutes at 425°F). When cool to the touch, slice or peel off the skin. Mince the peach and mix into a baby-sized serving of quinoa (½ cup).

quinoa fruit salad

total time: 30 minutes

servings: 4

½ cup quinoa, rinsed well

2½ cups mixed fruit, chopped (berries, peaches, kiwi, mango, etc.)

In a medium saucepan, combine the quinoa and 1¼ cups of water. Bring to a boil, cover, and simmer for 15 minutes, or until all of the water is absorbed. Turn off the heat and let sit, covered, for 5 minutes to steam. Fluff with a fork, then pour into a medium bowl. To cool quickly, place in the freezer.

Next, prepare the fruit. When the quinoa is cold, stir the fruit in to combine. Serve immediately or cover and place in the refrigerator until you're ready to serve.

multigrain hot cereal

preparation time: 5 minutes

cook time: 20 minutes

½ cup quinoa, rinsed well

½ cup steel-cut oats

2 cups water

1 teaspoon ground flaxseed

milk, brown sugar, and dried fruit for serving

In a medium saucepan, combine the quinoa, oats, ground flax, and water. Bring to a boil, cover, and reduce heat to low. Cook until the liquid is absorbed, about 20 minutes.

Stir in a splash of milk for creaminess and enjoy as-is, or top with brown sugar and dried fruit.

quinoa salad

preparation time: 5 minutes

cook time: 20 minutes

leftovers: 2 servings

½ cup quinoa, rinsed well

1¼ cups vegetable stock

1¼ cups frozen, shelled edamame

1 cup chopped kale

½ red pepper, diced

In a large microwave-safe bowl, combine the quinoa and vegetable stock. Cover and microwave for 9 minutes. Then add the edamame, kale, and red pepper. Microwave for 2 more minutes, and then fluff with a fork.

wheat berries 🩺

Wheat berries are wheat seeds. Since they are unprocessed, they contain all of the edible parts of the grain, making them extremely nutritious. Wheat berries are packed with essential vitamins and nutrients, such as fiber, iron, vitamin E, and antioxidants. They are high in gluten, so be sure to avoid them if you have gluten sensitivity.

wheat berry baby food

START WITH ¼ cup wheat berry cereal or ½ cup wheat berries

1. prep

If making whole wheat berries, pour them into a colander and sort through the berries, throwing out any stones. Rinse under water.

2. cook

To make wheat berry cereal, bring 1 cup of water to a boil in a small saucepan. Reduce heat to low and slowly pour the cereal into the boiling water. Mix well and cook for 20 minutes, stirring often until thickened.

To cook whole wheat berries, bring 1¼ cups water to a boil, and then add the wheat berries. Cover and simmer for 1 hour, stirring occasionally until tender and chewy. Drain the berries in a strainer.

3. add mix-ins & serve

simply wheat berry cereal
7 months +

MIX-INS

1 tablespoons breast milk, formula, or water

Stir breast milk, formula, or water into the wheat berry cereal. If the cereal thickens before serving, add more liquid to make a creamy, soupy consistency.

date and wheat berry cereal
8 months +

MIX-INS

8 dried dates

1 tablespoons breast milk, formula, or date cooking water

Plump the dates by placing them in a bowl and covering them with hot water. Let them sit for 5–10 minutes, or until plump. Use a slotted spoon to remove the dates (save the cooking water). Then slice and remove the seed from inside each date. Place the plumped dates and wheat berries, and breast milk, formula, or cooking water in a food processor and puree until smooth.

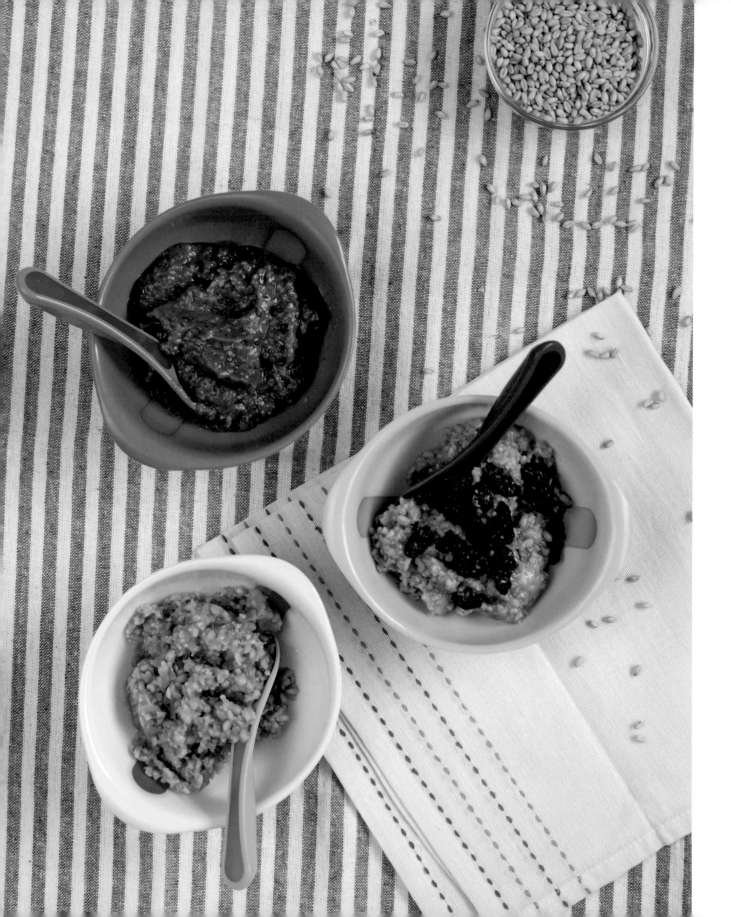

black bean and wheat berry puree

9 months +

MIX-INS

½ **cup black beans, cooked**

⅓ **cup breast milk, formula, or water**

Puree the wheat berries and black beans and breast milk, formula, or water in a blender to make a soft, lumpy puree.

apple wheat berries

10 months +

MIX-INS

2 **apples, peeled and chopped**

Cook the apples until tender (microwave for 3–4 minutes, steam for 12 minutes, or bake for 15 minutes at 375°F). Puree the apples and wheat berries in a blender to create a lumpy puree.

carrot, mango, apple, and wheat berries

11 months +

MIX-INS

¼ **cup chopped mango**

¼ **cup baby carrots**

¼ **cup peeled and chopped apple**

Cook the apple and carrots until tender (microwave for 3 minutes or steam for 7 minutes). Place the wheat berries, mango, carrots, and apple in a blender and pulse to finely dice.

raspberry-banana wheat berries

12 months +

MIX-INS

¾ **cup diced raspberries**

¼ **cup banana slices**

Puree all of the ingredients together, adding 3 tablespoons breast milk, formula, or water to make a soft, lumpy cereal, or mix the raspberries and bananas into the wheat berries and serve as finger food.

(facing page, clockwise from top)
date and wheat berry cereal;
raspberry-banana wheat berries;
carrot, mango, apple, and wheat berries

big batch of wheat berries

total time: 1 hour

makes: 4½ cups

As new parents, we are always looking for meals that are healthy and quick. Wheat berries are the perfect food for batch cooking. Make a big batch of them and eat throughout week.

7 cups water

2 cups wheat berries

½ teaspoon salt

Bring the water to a boil in a large saucepan, and then stir in the wheat berries and salt. Cover and cook for 1 hour, or until tender and chewy.

Drain the wheat berries in a strainer. Use right away, store in the refrigerator, or freeze for up to a month.

raspberry–banana wheat berry porridge

total time: 5 minutes

2 cups cooked wheat berries

⅓ cup milk

1 banana, peeled

½ cup raspberries

Place the wheat berries and milk in a large microwave-safe bowl and cook for 2 minutes.

Place the wheat berries, milk, and banana in a blender and whirl until smooth. Scoop the porridge into a bowl and top with raspberries.

mediterranean wheat berry salad

preparation time: 15 minutes

chill time: 30 minutes

2 cups cooked wheat berries, cold

½ cup chopped cucumber

¼ cup black olives

¼ cup crumbled feta

3 tablespoons balsamic dressing

In a large bowl, stir the wheat berries, cucumber, and olives together. Mix in the dressing, and then gently stir in the feta. Season to taste with salt and pepper.

Chill for 30 minutes to allow all the flavors to come together before serving (if you can wait that long!).

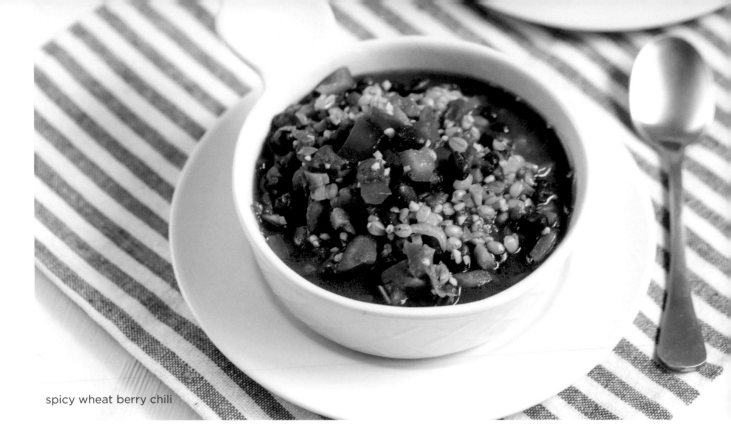

spicy wheat berry chili

spicy wheat berry chili

preparation: 10 minutes

cook time: 20 minutes

leftovers: 2 meals

As the name suggests, this chili is quite spicy! Reduce the amount of chili powder by half if you prefer a milder flavor.

2 tablespoons olive oil

½ cup onion, diced

½ red bell pepper, diced

1 jalapeño pepper, seeded and sliced

2 garlic cloves, minced

1 (15-ounce) can black beans, drained

1 (14-ounce) can diced tomatoes

1 cup cooked wheat berries

1 cup vegetable broth

1 teaspoon chili powder

1 teaspoon cumin

Heat the olive oil in a large skillet. Then add the onions, red peppers, jalapeños, and garlic. Cook until tender-crisp, about 7 minutes.

Meanwhile, heat the broth in the microwave for 1–2 minutes, or until hot.

Add the beans, tomatoes, cooked wheat berries, broth, and spices to the skillet and bring to a boil. Then reduce the heat and simmer for 10 minutes. Season to taste with salt and pepper.

Serve the chili piping hot in a serving bowl or over a baked potato. Top with cheddar cheese and sour cream if desired.

extras

how to make baby's first puree

1 Choose a fruit, vegetable, or protein suitable for your baby's age, and cook it if necessary.

2 Place in a blender and puree until completely smooth.

3 Add breast milk, formula, or water if necessary to create a smooth and soupy consistency.

4 Cool and serve!

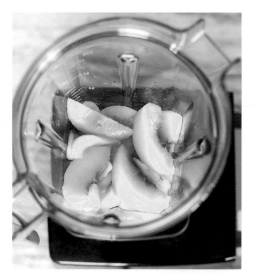

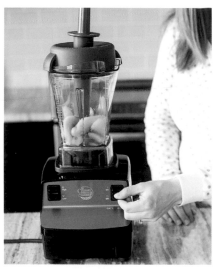

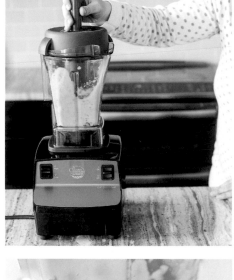

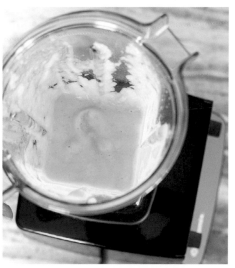

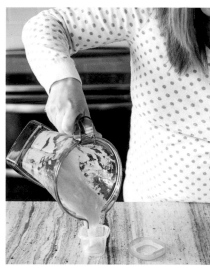

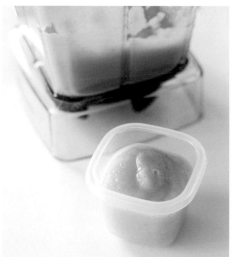

guide for making homemade infant cereal

You can easily make your own infant cereal at home using grains that are already in your pantry. Not only is this much less expensive than buying infant cereal at the store, but it can also be the more nutritious option.

how to make your own infant cereal

¼–2 cups uncooked grain (such as oats, wheat, or brown rice)

1 Place up to 2 cups grain into the coffee grinder, blender, or grain mill container, then secure with the lid.

2 Grind until the grain is uniformly ground into a powdery cereal.

3 You may want to stop and give the container a toss or stir with a spoon to make sure the whole batch gets evenly ground.

4 Pour into an airtight container or plastic bag. Then label with the name and date. Ground grains last up to 3 months in a cool pantry or freezer.

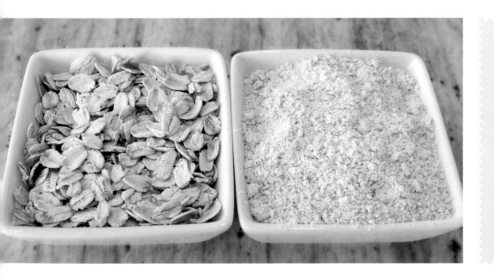

tools for grinding grains

- coffee grinder
- blender or food processor that can grinds grains
- grain mill or mixer with a grain mill attachment

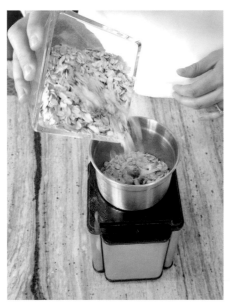
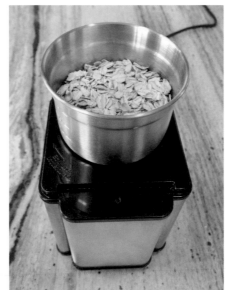
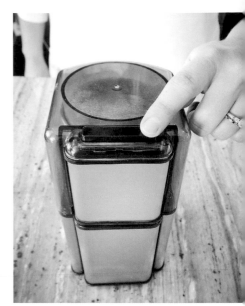

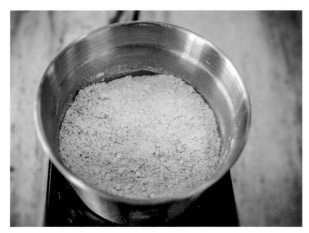

grains that make tasty cereal

* barley
* brown rice
* buckwheat
* bulgur
* millet
* oats
* quinoa
* wheat berries

gluten-free whole grains

* brown rice
* buckwheat
* millet
* oats
* quinoa

2 ways to cook homemade infant cereal

traditional method

1. In a saucepan, heat water to boiling. Reduce the temperature to low, and slowly add cereal, stirring constantly to prevent lumping. If you can't stir constantly because you're holding your baby, then just slowly add the cereal in a steady stream, then briskly stir with a whisk to break up any clumps.

2. Cover, leaving a small air vent, and simmer until the cereal is tender, stirring occasionally. Stir in breast milk or formula to add creaminess and thin the consistency. As with all food, cool before serving to baby.

note: As the cereal sits, it will thicken. Add additional liquid if you need to just before serving.

overnight stovetop method

1. Just before bed, bring the appropriate amount of water to a boil. Then mix in the infant cereal.

2. Turn off the burner, cover, and let the cereal soak overnight. When you awake in the morning, the cereal will be ready to eat cold. If you want to serve it warm, simply turn the burner on low to heat.

helpful hints

* Combine grains for variety.

* Stir in breast milk, formula, or yogurt to make the cereal creamy.

* Store uncooked infant cereal in the freezer for freshness.

* If the cereal hasn't thickened by the recommended amount of time, increase the heat and continue cooking until thick.

cooking guide for infant cereal

infant cereal	amount	water	cooking time	cereal yield
barley	½ cup	2 cups	20 minutes	1½ cups
brown rice	½ cup	2 cups	15 minutes	1 ¾ cups
buckwheat	½ cup	2 cups	10 minutes	1 ⅔ cups
bulgur	⅔ cup	2½ cups	7 minutes	1½ cups
millet	½ cup	2 cups	10 minutes	1½ cups
oats	½ cup	2 cups	20 minutes	1½ cups
quinoa	½ cup	1 ½ cups	12 minutes	1½ cups
wheat berries	½ cup	2 cups	20 minutes	1⅓ cups

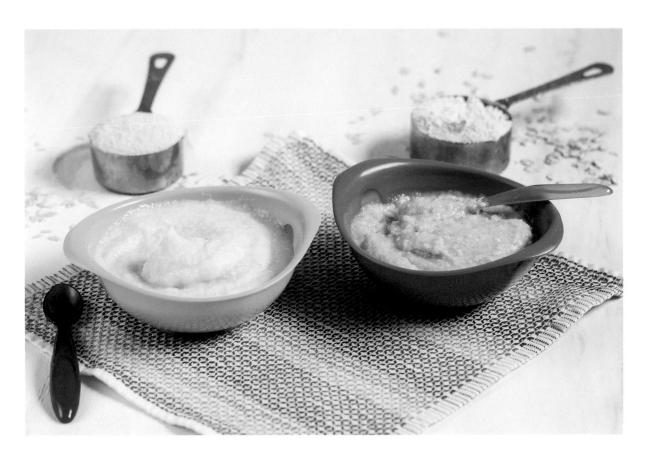

2 ways to cook homemade infant cereal

age guide for introducing solid foods

6 months

apples	pears	chicken	turkey
avocado	carrots	low-mercury fish	oats
bananas	beef	brown rice	sweet potatoes

7 months

peaches	plums	barley	green beans
figs	prunes	millet	
plantains	squash	wheat berries	

8 months

blueberries	brussels sprouts	tofu	bulgur
kiwifruits	cauliflower	edamame	quinoa
mangoes	egg yolk	buckwheat	

9 months

honeydew and cantaloupe	peas	pork	full-fat cottage cheese
papayas	broccoli	russet potatoes	unsweetened whole milk yogurt
asparagus	prepared beans	chia seeds	

10 months

spinach	flaxseed	hard cheese, ie. cheddar	
kale	wheat germ		

11 months

pineapples	turnips		

baby's food diary

first food: ....

.... date: ....

baby's reaction to trying solid food: ....

....

....

first finger food: ....

.... date: ....

favorite fruits: ....

....

favorite vegetables: ....

....

favorite meats: ....

....

favorite grains: ....

....

new foods and textures that baby tried this month

6 months: ....

....

7 months: ....

....

8 months: ....

....

9 months: ....

....

10 months: ....

....

11 months: ....

....

12 months: ....

....

food allergy journal

Writing down which foods your child reacts to makes it much easier to keep track of food allergies. Sometimes when our little ones have reactions to certain foods, we remember to avoid them for a while, but forget down the line. Save yourself the trial and error, and jot down any food allergy symptoms as soon as they appear.

suspected allergenic food: .... date tried:..................................

reaction: ....

....

....

suspected allergenic food: .... date tried:..................................

reaction: ....

....

....

suspected allergenic food: .... date tried:..................................

reaction: ....

....

....

suspected allergenic food: .... date tried:..................................

reaction: ....

....

notes

1. Ada L. García et al., "Nutritional content of infant commercial weaning foods in the UK," *Archives of Disease in Childhood* 98, no. 10 (2013): 793. doi: 10.1136/archdischild-2012-303386.
2. American Academy of Family Physicians, "Breastfeeding (Policy Statement)," accessed February 6, 2017, http://www.aafp.org/about/policies/all/breastfeeding.html.
3. Michael Crocetti, Robert A. Dudas, and Scott D. Krugman, "Parental Beliefs and Practices Regarding Early Introduction of Solid Foods to Their Children," *Clinical Pediatrics* 46, no. 6 (2004): 541–47. doi: 10.1177/000992280404300606.
4. Alice A. Kuo et al., "Introduction of Solid Food to Young Infants," *Maternal and Child Health Journal* 15, no. 8 (2011): 1185–94. doi: 10.1007/s10995-010-0669-5.
5. United States Department of Agriculture, "Infant Nutrition and Feeding: A Guide for Use in the WIC and CSF Programs," USDA, last modified March 2009, accessed February 6, 2017, https://wicworks.fns.usda.gov/wicworks/Topics/FG/CompleteIFG.pdf.
6. Kuo et al., "Introduction of Solid Food to Young Infants."
7. American Academy of Pediatrics "Promoting Healthy Nutrition," Bright Futures, accessed February 6, 2017, https://brightfutures.aap.org/Bright%20Futures%20Documents/6-Promoting_Healthy_Nutrition.pdf.
8. "Introducing Solid Foods: 6 Reasons Why You Should Wait to Introduce Solid Food to Your Baby," AskDrSears.com, accessed February 6, 2017, http://www.askdrsears.com/topics/feeding-eating/feeding-infants-toddlers/starting-solids/introducing-solid-foods.
9. Kerri Wachter, "Rice cereal can wait, let them eat meat first: AAP committee has changes in mind," *Pediatric News*, November 1, 2009, http://www.mdedge.com/internalmedicinenews/404 (site discontinued).
10. Ibid.
11. National Institute of Diabetes and Digestive and Kidney Diseases, "Foodborne Illnesses," U.S. Department of Health and Human Services, accessed December 8, 2016, https://www.niddk.nih.gov/health-information/digestive-diseases/foodborne-illnesses#4.
12. United States Department of Agriculture, "Organic Production & Handling Standards," USDA, last modified November 2016, accessed February 6, 2017, https://www.ams.usda.gov/publications/content/organic-production-handling-standards.
13. American Academy of Pediatrics, "Policy Statement: Pesticide Exposure in Children," *Pediatrics* 130, no. 6 (2012): e1757–63. doi: 10.1542/peds.2012-2757.
14. U.S. Department of Health and Human Services, *Reducing Environmental Cancer Risk: What We Can Do Now.* National Institutes of Health, National Cancer Institute, last modified April 2010, accessed February 6, 2017, https://deainfo.nci.nih.gov/advisory/pcp/annualReports/pcp08-09rpt/PCP_Report_08-09_508.pdf.
15. American Academy of Pediatrics, "Food Allergy Reactions: How do I know if my child has a food allergy?" last modified November 2010, accessed February 6, 2017, https://www.healthychildren.org/English/ages-stages/baby/feeding-nutrition/Pages/Food-Allergy-Reactions.aspx.
16. "Eat the Peach, Not the Pesticide," *Consumer Reports*, March 19, 2015, accessed February 6, 2017, http://www.consumerreports.org/cro/health/natural-health/pesticides/index.htm.
17. Melissa Wagner-Schuman et al., "Association of pyrethroid pesticide exposure with attention-deficit/hyperactivity disorder in a nationally representative sample of U.S. children," *Environmental Health* 14, no. 44 (2015). doi: 10.1186/s12940-015-0030-y.

18. Brenda Eskenazi et al., "Organophosphate Pesticide Exposure and Neurodevelopment in Young Mexican-American Children," *Environmental Health Perspectives* 115, no. 2 (2007): 792–98. doi: 10.1289/ehp.9828.

19. Maryse F. Bouchard et al., "Prenatal Exposure to Organophosphate Pesticides and IQ in 7-Year-Old Children," *Environmental Health Perspectives* 119, no. 8 (2011): 1189–95. doi: 10.1289/ehp.1003185.

20. "Eat the Peach, Not the Pesticide."

21. Center for Ecogenetics & Environmental Health, "Fast Facts about Health Risks of Pesticides in Food," University of Washington, last modified January 2013, accessed February 6, 2017, https://depts.washington.edu/ceeh/downloads/FF_Pesticides.pdf.

22. Environmental Working Group, "Executive Summary: EWG's 2016 Shopper's Guide to Pesticides in Produce™," accessed February 6, 2017, https://www.ewg.org/foodnews/summary.php.

23. Chensheng Lu et al., "Organic Diets Significantly Lower Children's Dietary Exposure to Organophosphorus Pesticides," *Environmental Health Perspectives* 114, no 2: (2006) 260–63. doi: 10.1289/ehp.8418.

24. George Du Toit et al., "Effect of Avoidance on Peanut Allergy after Early Peanut Consumption," *The New England Journal of Medicine* 374 (2016): 1435–43. doi: 10.1056/NEJMoa1514209.

25. Kuo et al., "Introduction of Solid Food to Young Infants."

26. Katie A. Loth et al., "Food-Related Parenting Practices and Adolescent Weight Status: A Population-Based Study," *Pediatrics* 131, no. 5 (2013): e1443–50. doi: 10.1542/peds.2012-3073.

27. Mary Kay Fox et al., "Average Portions of Foods Commonly Eaten by Infants and Toddlers in the United States." *Journal of the American Dietetic Association* 106, no. 1 (2006): s66–76. doi: 10.1016/j.jada.2005.09.042.

28. Erik Lykke Mortensen, Kim Fleisher Michaelsem, and Stephanie A. Sanders, "The Association Between Duration of Breastfeeding and Adult Intelligence," *JAMA* 287, no. 18 (2002): 2365–71. doi:10.1001/jama.287.18.2365.

29. World Health Organization, "Exclusive breastfeeding," accessed February 6, 2017, http://www.who.int/nutrition/topics/exclusive_breastfeeding/en.

30. García et al., "Nutritional content of infant commercial weaning foods in the UK."

31. World Health Organization, "Exclusive breastfeeding."

32. "Adopting optimal feeding practices is fundamental to a child's survival, growth and development, but too few children benefit," UNICEF, last modified October 2016, accessed February 6, 2017, http://data.unicef.org/topic/nutrition/infant-and-young-child-feeding/.

33. Environmental Working Group, "Executive Summary: EWG's 2016 Shopper's Guide to Pesticides in Produce™."

34. United States Department of Agriculture, "Eating Fish While You Are Pregnant or Breastfeeding," USDA, ChooseMyPlate.gov, last modified January 26, 2017, accessed February 6, 2017, https://www.choosemyplate.gov/moms-food-safety-fish.

works consulted

Allen, Minako Takamiya, and Leonard S. Levy. "Parkinson's disease and pesticide exposure—a new assessment." *Critical Reviews in Toxicology* 43, no. 6 (2013): 515–34. doi: 10.3109/10408444.2013.798719.

American Academy of Family Physicians. "Breastfeeding (Policy Statement)." AAFP. http://www.aafp.org/about/policies/all/breastfeeding.html.

American Academy of Pediatrics. "Aerial Spraying to Combat Mosquitos Linked to Increased Risk of Autism in Children." April 30, 2016. https://www.aap.org/en-us/about-the-aap/aap-press-room/pages/Aerial-Spraying-to-Combat-Mosquitos-Linked-to-Increased-Risk-of-Autism-in-Children.aspx.

American Academy of Pediatrics. "Food Allergy Reactions: How do I know if my child has a food allergy?" AAFP. https://www.healthychildren.org/English/ages-stages/baby/feeding-nutrition/Pages/Food-Allergy-Reactions.aspx.

American Academy of Pediatrics. "Policy Statement: Breastfeeding and the Use of Human Milk." *Pediatrics* 129, no. 3 (2012): e827–41. doi: 10.1086/ahr.113.3.752.

American Academy of Pediatrics. "Policy Statement: Pesticide Exposure in Children." *Pediatrics* 130, no. 6 (2012): e1757–63. doi: 10.1542/peds.2012-2757.

American Academy of Pediatrics. "Promoting Healthy Nutrition." Bright Futures—AAP. https://brightfutures.aap.org/Bright%20Futures%20Documents/6-Promoting_Healthy_Nutrition.pdf.

Bouchard, Maryse F., Jonathan Chevrier, Kim G. Harley, Katherine Kogut, Michelle Vedar, Norma Calderon, Celina Trujillo, et al. "Prenatal Exposure to Organophosphate Pesticides and IQ in 7-Year-Old Children." *Environmental Health Perspectives* 119, no. 8 (2011): 1189–95. doi: 10.1289/ehp.1003185.

Center for Ecogenetics & Environmental Health, University of Washington. "Fast Facts about Health Risks of Pesticides in Food." https://depts.washington.edu/ceeh/downloads/FF_Pesticides.pdf.

Crocetti, Michael, Robert A. Dudas, and Scott D. Krugman. "Parental Beliefs and Practices Regarding Early Introduction of Solid Foods to Their Children." *Clinical Pediatrics* 46, no. 6 (2004): 541–47. doi: 10.1177/000992280404300606.

Curl, Cynthia L., Shirley A. A. Beresford, Richard A Fenske, Annette L. Fitzpatrick, Chensheng Lu, Jennifer A. Nettleton, and Joel D. Kaufman. "Estimating Pesticide Exposure from Dietary Intake and Organic Food Choices: The Multi-Ethnic Study of Atherosclerosis (MESA)." *Environmental Health Perspectives* 123, no. 5 (2014): 475–83. doi: 10.1289/ehp.1408197.

Du Toit, George, Peter H. Sayre, Graham Roberts, Michelle L. Sever, Kaitie Lawson, Henry T. Bahnson, Helen A. Brough et al. "Effect of Avoidance on Peanut Allergy after Early Peanut Consumption." *The New England Journal of Medicine* 374 (2016): 1435–43. doi: 10.1056/NEJMoa1514209.

"Eat the Peach, Not the Pesticide." *Consumer Reports*, March 19, 2015. http://www.consumerreports.org/cro/health/natural-health/pesticides/index.htm.

Environmental Working Group. "Executive Summary: EWG's 2016 Shopper's Guide to Pesticides in Produce™." https://www.ewg.org/foodnews/summary.php.

Eskenazi, Brenda, Amy R. Marks, Asa Bradman, Kim Harley, Dana B. Barr, Caroline Johnson, Norma Morga, and Nicholas P. Jewell. "Organophosphate Pesticide Exposure and Neurodevelopment in Young Mexican-American Children." *Environmental Health Perspectives* 115, no. 2 (2007): 792–98. doi: 10.1289/ehp.9828.

Fox, Mary Kay, Kathleen Reidy, Vatsala Karwe, and Paula Zeigler. "Average Portions of Foods Commonly Eaten by Infants and Toddlers in the United States." *Journal of the American Dietetic Association* 106, no. 1 (2006): s66–76.
doi: 10.1016/j.jada.2005.09.042.

García, Ada L., Sarah Raza, Alison Parrett, and Charlotte M. Wright. "Nutritional content of infant commercial weaning foods in the UK." *Archives of Disease in Childhood* 98, no. 10 (2013): 793. doi: 10.1136/archdischild-2012-303386.

"Introducing Solid Foods: 6 Reasons Why You Should Wait to Introduce Solid Food to Your Baby." AskDrSears.com. http://www.askdrsears.com/topics/feeding-eating/feeding-infants-toddlers/starting-solids/introducing-solid-foods.

Kuo, Alice A., Moira Inkelas, Wendelin M. Slusser, Molly Maidenberg, and Neal Halfon. "Introduction of Solid Food to Young Infants." *Maternal and Child Health Journal* 15, no. 8 (2011): 1185–94. doi: 10.1007/s10995-010-0669-5.

Loth, Katie A., Richard F. MacLehose, Jayne A. Fulkerson, Scott Cross, and Dianne Neumark-Sztainer. "Food-Related Parenting Practices and Adolescent Weight Status: A Population-Based Study." *Pediatrics* 131, no. 5 (2013): e1443–50. doi: 10.1542/peds.2012-3073.

Lu, Chensheng, Kathryn Toepel, Rene Irish, Richard A. Fensky, Dana B. Barr, and Roberto Bravo. "Organic Diets Significantly Lower Children's Dietary Exposure to Organophosphorus Pesticides." *Environmental Health Perspectives* 114, no 2: (2006) 260–63. doi: 10.1289/ehp.8418.

Mortensen, Erik Lykke, Kim Fleisher Michaelsem, and Stephanie A. Sanders. "The Association Between Duration of Breastfeeding and Adult Intelligence." *JAMA* 287, no. 18 (2002): 2365–71. doi:10.1001/jama.287.18.2365.

National Institute of Diabetes and Digestive and Kidney Diseases. "Foodborne Illnesses." U.S. Department of Health and Human Services. https://www.niddk.nih.gov/health-information/digestive-diseases/foodborne-illnesses#4.

Norris, Jill M., Katherine Barriga, Georgeanna Klingensmoth, Michelle Hoffman, Goerge S. Eisenbarth, Henry A. Erlich, and Marian Rewers. "Timing of Initial Cereal Exposure in Infancy and Risk of Islet Autoimmunity." *JAMA* 290, no. 13 (2003): 1713–20. doi: 10.1001/jama.290.13.1713.

Oates, Liza, Marc Cohen, Lesley Braun, Adrian Schembri, and Rilka Taskova. "Reduction in urinary organophosphate pesticide metabolites in adults after a week-long organic diet." *Environmental Research* 132 (2014): 105–11. doi: 10.1016/j.envres.2014.03.021.

Rauh, Virginia A., Robin Garfinkel, Frederica P. Perera, Howard F. Andrews, Lori Hoepner, Dana B. Barr, Ralph Whitehead et al. " Impact of Prenatal Chlorpyrifos Exposure on Neurodevelopment in the First 3 Years of Life Among Inner-City Children." *Pediatrics* 118, no. 6 (2006): e1845–59. http://pediatrics.aappublications.org/content/118/6/e1845.

UNICEF. "Adopting optimal feeding practices is fundamental to a child's survival, growth and development, but too few children benefit." http://data.unicef.org/topic/nutrition/infant-and-young-child-feeding/.

United States Department of Agriculture. "Eating Fish While You Are Pregnant or Breastfeeding." USDA, ChooseMyPlate.gov. https://www.choosemyplate.gov/moms-food-safety-fish.

United States Department of Agriculture. "Infant Nutrition and Feeding: A Guide for Use in the WIC and CSF Programs." USDA. https://wicworks.fns.usda.gov/wicworks/Topics/FG/CompleteIFG.pdf.

United States Department of Agriculture. "Organic Production & Handling Standards." USDA. https://www.ams.usda.gov/publications/content/organic-production-handling-standards.

United States Department of Health and Human Services. *Reducing Environmental Cancer Risk: What We Can Do Now.* USDHHS/NIH/NIC. https://deainfo.nci.nih.gov/advisory/pcp/annualReports/pcp08-09rpt/PCP_Report_08-09_508.pdf.

index

happy tummies

happy tummies

To my husband, who inspires me to dream big every day.

You have encouraged me every step of the way. Without your support,
my idea for this book may have only amounted to a few notes jotted on
a hotel sticky pad, and a bunch of unfinished documents on my computer.
Thank you for believing in me and in my ideas, and for taking care
of our little one while I wrote and tested recipes.

Thank you for all of your love and continued support. You are amazing!

*And to my little ones, whose laughs light up my soul
and whose smiles are contagious.*

Thank you for taste-testing so many of my recipes, and for inspiring me
to be a better mother each and every day.

I love you guys

Bright Ideas Publishing
3450 N. Triumph Blvd. Suite 102
Lehi, UT 84043, USA
530-436-5245
www.happytummiescookbook.com
www.folcik.com

Happy Tummies
Conceived and produced by Karen Folcik

Library of Congress Cataloging-in-Publication Data is available upon request.

ISBN 978-0-692-89141-4

Bright Ideas Publishing is a division of Folcik Enterprises, LLC.

Folcik Enterprises
CEO and Principal Mike Folcik
AUTHOR: Karen Folcik, MSW
FEATURED NUTRITIONIST: Cassandra Edwards, MS, RDN/LD
FOOD PHOTOGRAPHER AND FOOD STYLIST: Tiffany Anderson
INFANT PHOTOGRAPHER: Shauna Purser
ADDITIONAL PHOTOGRAPHY AND PHOTO EDITING: Chi Mei Tracy Omae
EDITED BY: NY Book Editors
BOOK DESIGN BY: Vertigo Design, Inc.

PRINTED AND BOUND IN THE UNITED STATES OF AMERICA

Karen is a wife and mom to a clever three-year-old boy, and a happy baby boy. She enjoys hiking, biking, and picnicking with her family, and is constantly surprised at the journey of motherhood. Before motherhood, Karen studied psychology at Florida Gulf Coast University, and earned her MSW from Columbia University. She counseled kids and families as a practicing social worker. Karen hopes that this book is a blessing for every new mother that chooses to read it. A Connecticut native, Karen and her family now call Utah Valley home.

Cassandra is a practicing nutrition educator and registered dietitian. She has her own private practice, where she offers one-on-one nutrition counseling to new moms and classes on how to make your own baby food. She has also worked at Women, Infants and Children (WIC) teaching nutrition classes and writing handbooks that teach parents how to feed their children. Most importantly, Cassandra is a mother of two, and she eagerly fed them both homemade baby food.

Tiffany Anderson is a food photographer who loves capturing beautiful food. She is passionate about healthy eating and loves to share nutritious meals with others. Tiffany enjoys living in Utah and spends most of her time exploring in the mountains with her family.